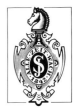

M.E. Müller S. Nazarian P. Koch J. Schatzker

The Comprehensive
Classification of Fractures
of Long Bones

With the Collaboration of Urs Heim

With 93 Figures, Mostly in Colour

Springer-Verlag
Berlin Heidelberg New York
London Paris Tokyo
Hong Kong Barcelona

Prof. Dr. med. Maurice E. Müller
Fondation Maurice E. Müller
Murtenstr. 35
CH-3001 Bern

Prof. Dr. med. Serge Nazarian
Service d'Orthopédie, Traumatologie
et Chirurgie Vertébrale
Hôpital de la Conception
147, Boulevard Baille
F-13004 Marseille

Collaborator:
PD Dr. med. Urs F. A. Heim
AO-International
Balderstr. 30
CH-3007 Bern

Dr. med. Peter Koch
Fondation Maurice E. Müller
Documentation Centre
Murtenstr. 35
CH-3001 Bern

Joseph Schatzker, M.D., F.R.C.S.(C)
Chief of Orthopaedics
Sunnybrook Medical Centre
2075 Bayview Avenue
Toronto, Ontario M4N 3M5, Canada

ISBN 3-540-18165-2 Springer-Verlag Berlin Heidelberg New York Tokyo
ISBN 0-387-18165-2 Springer-Verlag New York Berlin Heidelberg Tokyo
ISBN 4-431-18165-2 Springer-Verlag Tokyo Berlin Heidelberg New York

Library of Congress Cataloging-in-Publication Data. The Comprehensive classification of fractures of long bones/ M.E. Müller ... [et al.] with the collaboration of Urs Heim. p. cm. Includes bibliographical references. Includes index. ISBN 3-540-18165-2 (alk. paper).–ISBN 0-387-18165-2 (alk. paper) 1. Fractures–Classification. I. Müller, M.E. (Maurice Edmond), 1918– . [DNLM: 1. Fractures–classification. WE 15 C737] RD101.C7195 1990 617.1'5–dc20 DNLM/DLC 90-10033

Reproduction of the figures: Gustav Dreher GmbH, D-7000 Stuttgart
Printing and bookbinding: Druckhaus Beltz, D-6944 Hemsbach
2124/3130-543210 – Printed on acid-free paper

Preface to the English Edition

The history of the origin and development of the new Classification of Fractures was described in the preface to the French edition. The history of the acceptance of this new concept dates back to 1986, when the Swiss Association for the Study of the Problems of Internal Fixation (AO) accepted the new Classification of Fractures. In the same year, the Trustees of the AO/ASIF Foundation, at their annual meeting in Montreux, adopted the new AO Classification as the basis for fracture classification to be used in the planned third edition of the AO/ASIF Manual.

In August 1987, the French edition of *"The Comprehensive Classification of Fractures of Long Bones"* made its first appearance, coincident with the Congress of the International Society of Orthopaedic Surgery (SICOT) in Munich. This precipitated a great deal of interest in the subject. This interest persisted, so that in February of 1988 the President of SICOT, Sir Dennis Paterson, formed a "Presidential Commission for Documentation and Evaluation" with Maurice E. Müller as Chairman.

In the fall of 1987, Joseph Schatzker began the translation of the newly published book from French into English. His critical evaluation of our work, his great familiarity with fractures and his ability to formulate clear concise and creative concepts led to a revision of some of our ideas and clarification of others. We invited him to join us as a co-author and began, with his help, the difficult task of creating very precise definitions of terms for the new glossary, which became the basis for the subsequent translation. In the summer of 1988, we published a precis of the "AO Classification of Fractures" simultaneously in six languages. It became the basis for further discussion and evaluation of the work by the SICOT Commission, as well as by the Trustees of the AO Foundation.

Berne, February 1990

Maurice E. Müller
Serge Nazarian
Peter Koch
Joseph Schatzker

Preface to the French Edition

Around the beginning of 1970 it became apparent that there was a need to create a systematic orderly classification system of fractures of the whole skeleton. A review of the medical literature disclosed that many attempts had been made to classify fractures. All these classifications, however, were based on the involved segment. None attempted to present a **unified scheme** of classification of the whole skeleton. This book is an attempt to fulfill this need.

The AO/ASIF Documentation Centre in Berne has been an excellent resource for the study of the problem. Between the years 1958 and 1986 it accumulated an archive of more than one million X-rays. These represent more than 150,000 of operatively treated fractures. The wealth of information which we had at our disposal through the collected and documented cases greatly simplified our task of comparing our methods of classification with those based on anatomical areas and their lesions. We were in the position to identify some significant common features which were valid not only for the diaphyseal but also for the articular fractures.

In the summer of 1977, while I was still the chief of the Orthopaedic Department at the University of Berne, we decided to create a general classification of all fractures which would be used by the whole AO group. In order to accomplish this task, I assigned to my senior residents and residents the responsibility of taking 100 fractures of each specific bony segment and then segregating them into 9 groups and 3 subgroups. I should like to single out and express my gratitude to the folowing participants in this project: Reinhold Ganz, Bruno Noesberger, Peter Bamert, Hans-Ueli Stäubli, Andreas Lehmann, Vasiliji Mustur, Michael Sturzenegger, Peter Engelhardt, Guido Mäder, and Gontran Sennwald. Other co-workers used this opportunity to submit their study of a particular bony segment either as a thesis for a postgraduate degree or for publication. Thus Roland Jakob came to study the proximal humerus, Diego Fernandez the distal radius, Eric Jeanmaire the fractures of the femoral neck, Rudolf Johner the tibial shaft, and Engelbert Gross the diaphysis of the radius and ulna. These studies led to the creation of a temporary classification which was subsequently adopted by the AO group and used for a period of 9 years. This afforded the AO Documentation Centre a unique opportunity to study this classification and evaluate all its advantages and disadvantages.

In 1980 we began a collaboration with Dr. Serge Nazarian, a French surgeon and anatomist who is also a gifted didactic and critical thinker. We compared the classifications and the cases published in the world literature between the years 1977 and 1979 with those classified according to the AO classification and documented in the AO Documentation Centre. As the next step, in collaboration with Dr. Peter Koch we analyzed, more than 15,000 fully documented fractures which came from the following clinics: Basle (M. Allgöwer and F. Harder), Berne (M.E. Müller and R. Ganz), St-Gall (B.G. Weber), Chur (Th. Rüedi), Interlaken (B. Noesberger) and Davos

(P. Matter). In this analysis the following collaborators must be distinguished for their effort: Peter Koch (femoral fractures), Hans-Peter Madl (fractures of the proximal tibia), Frank Möller (distal humerus), and Peter Witschger (tibial diaphysis). Many ideas were also contributed by the AO pioneers such as Martin Allgöwer, Thomas Rüedi, and Peter Matter. We must make particular mention of Urs Heim because the ideas which he published in his book *"Internal fixation of small fractures. Techniques recommended by the AO-ASIF group"* and in his book about the distal tibia profoundly influenced our concepts about the delineation of the end segments of the long bones and about the classification of the fractures of the distal tibia.

The AO Group has now fully adopted the following principle of documentation: the codification of the fractures is accomplished with the help of 2 numbers which give the anatomical localization of the lesion, and 1 letter and 2 numbers which express the morphologic characteristics. The aim of this book is to demonstrate how one can establish a precise diagnosis with the help of 3 questions, each of which has 3 possible answers, so that the surgeon will be aided in selecting the best possible treatment. In order to draw attention to the severity of the injury we have coloured more than 500 schematic drawings either in green, orange, or red. These colours should denote in the same way as the letters A, B, and C the severity of the injury, that is, the difficulties one may encounter in operative treatment, the likelihood of complications, and the prognosis.

We are particularly indebted to Mrs. Eleonore Moosberger, the secretary of the M.E. Müller Foundation, for her patient and tireless collaboration in the project. She was always there when we needed her and not only did she pull the manuscript together with her computer, but she also prepared it perfectly for direct transmission to the printer. We wish to thank also all our medical collaborators, particularly Urs Heim for his constructive criticism, and Peter Koch for his willingness and extraordinary precision. We are also grateful to our artist Klaus Oberli for his brilliant graphic representation of our ideas.

Our collaboration with the representatives of Springer-Verlag was most agreeable. Their competence in and friendliness towards the project enabled the publisher to produce a book which is of excellent quality. For this we are very grateful.

Berne, July 1, 1987   Maurice E. Müller
SICOT, August 20, 1987

Collaborators on specific segments:

11-   Humerus Proximal   Roland Jakob, M.D.
University Clinic of Orthopaedic Surgery, Inselspital, CH-3010 Bern

13-   Humerus Distal   Frank Möller, M.D.
University Clinic for Orthopaedics, Siegmund-Freud-Strasse 25, D-5300 Bonn-Venusberg

23-   Radius/Ulna Distal   Diego L. Fernandez, M.D.
Department of Traumatology, Kantonsspital, CH-5000 Aarau

42-   Tibia Diaphysis   Pierre Witschger, M.D.
University Clinic for Orthopaedic Surgery, Inselspital, CH-3010 Bern

Addresses of collaborators on specific segments:

51-53 Aebi Max, M.D., University Clinic of Orthopaedic Surgery, Inselspital, CH-3010 Bern

53-   Magerl Fritz, M.D., Chairman Service of Orthopaedic Surgery and Traumatology,
Kantonsspital, CH-9009 St. Gallen

61-   Isler Balz, M.D., Department of Orthopaedic Surgery, Kantonsspital , CH-8401 Winterthur
Tile Marvin, M.D., Chief Orthopaedic Surgeon, Sunnybrook Medical Centre, 2075 Bayview
Avenue, CND-Toronto, Ont. M4N 3M5

62-   Letournel Emile, M.D., Professor of Orthopaedic Surgery and Traumatology,
Centre Médico-chirurgical de la Porte de Choisy, Service d´Orthopédie et de Traumatologie,
15, ave. de la Porte de Choisy, F-75634 Paris Cedex 13
Mast Jeffrey W., M.D., c/o Teitge Orthopaedics, 4050 East Twelve Mile Road, Suite 110,
USA-Warren, MI 48092,
Matta Joel M., M.D., Department of Orthopaedics , Pelvis and Hip Reconstruction, Suite 600,
637 South Lucas Street, USA-Los Angeles, CA 90017

8   Hansen Sigward T.Jr., M.D., Department of Orthopaedics, One West Highland Drive,
USA-Seattle, WA 98119
Jorda Eduardo, M.D., 18, Paseo Mallorca, Palma de Mallorca, Espagne

Table of Contents

Special Section, Long Bones

Introduction

In deciding on the type of treatment for a specific fracture, the surgeon must use as a basis, to a lesser or greater degree, the morphological features of the fracture. We felt therefore that if a classification were to be useful for a surgeon as a guide to treatment, it had to embody the essence of these morphological features. Thus we began with an analysis of the different bones in order to establish some common features shared not only by the fractures of the diaphyses but also by the fractures of the end segments, that is the metaphyses and epiphyses.

As the next step in the development of our classification, we arranged the fractures in an increasing order of severity. For us the term "severity" implies anticipated difficulties of treatment, the likely complications, and the prognosis.

Once this was accomplished, we faced two further problems. We had to establish a suitable terminology and find a practical method of carrying out our classification.

In creating the new terminology, we made certain that the terms we chose would define similar injuries irrespective of their anatomical location. This unified terminology together with the exact definitions of all terms is to be found at the end of this book in the "Glossary".

The classification method was a more complex problem. An acceptable system had to be based on an alpha-numerical code which would permit the localization and morphological characterization of every fracture. Furthermore, this code had to be structured in such a way that it could be entered directly into a computer for analysis. The system which we finally designed is similar to the classification which Linné developed for the classification of plants. Our system is, however, simpler and better suited for the data it deals with.

To use our system of classification one has to ask three questions, each of which has three possible answers. The answers allow one to classify the fracture and in this way define its inherent prognosis and therapeutic difficulties.

We began with an analysis of all the documented cases of fractures of the long bones. These are not only common, but also share many similarities, which greatly eased the task of their classification. The classification of fractures of the bones or groups of bones which comprise the remainder of the skeleton will be included in the next volume. These fractures are not only less common, but also much more difficult to classify. It is our intent, however, to retain the same uniform system of terminology and severity grading of the classification.

General Section

1. Principles of the Classification of Fractures

A classification is useful only if it considers the severity of the bone lesion and serves as a basis for treatment and for evaluation of the results.

To classify a fracture one must know its **morphological characteristics** and its **location** . The **coding** of the morphology and the location must be simple and easy to memorize.

1.1 Morphological Characterization of a Fracture

The characterization of the morphology of the fracture (= bone lesion) is based on the fact that fractures of all bone segments are classified in 3 types which are divided into 3 groups and further subdivided into 3 subgroups. Thus, the **3 questions: 1. Which type? ... 2. Which group? ... 3. Which subgroup? ...** and the **3 possible answers** to each are the key to the morphological characterization of the fracture and to the classification.

The type is indicated by one of the 3 letters: **A, B,** or **C.** Each of the 3 types is divided into 3 groups which are given a number: **1, 2,** or **3.** This provides 9 groups (**A1, A2, A3 – B1, B2, B3 – C1, C2, C3**) for each bone segment. Each group is then further subdivided into 3 subgroups, denoted by a number: **.1, .2,** or **.3.**

In the classification the 9 groups are organized in order of **increasing severity**, based on their morphological complexity, the difficulty of treatment and their prognosis. The order of the colours green, orange and red, as well as the increasing darkness of the arrows, indicate the increasing severity. A1 indicates the simplest fracture with the best prognosis and C3 the most difficult with the worst prognosis. Once a surgeon has classified a fracture, he will have established its severity and thus obtained a guide to treatment.

If a fracture cannot be assigned to any of the groups, it is placed in a separate group **D1**. In such a case it is necessary to describe the fracture fully. Such fractures are extremely rare.

Fig. 1   **The scheme of the classification of fractures for each bone segment or each bone**

Types:	**A, B, C**		
Groups:	**A1, A2, A3**	**B1, B2, B3**	**C1, C2, C3**
Subgroups:	**.1, .2, .3**		

The **colours** green, orange, and red correspond in significance to those of a traffic signal. The sequence of the colours as well as the darkening of the arrows indicate the increasing severity of the fracture.

The small **squares**: the two first ones give the location (see p. 4); the next three give the morphological characteristics of the fracture.

4

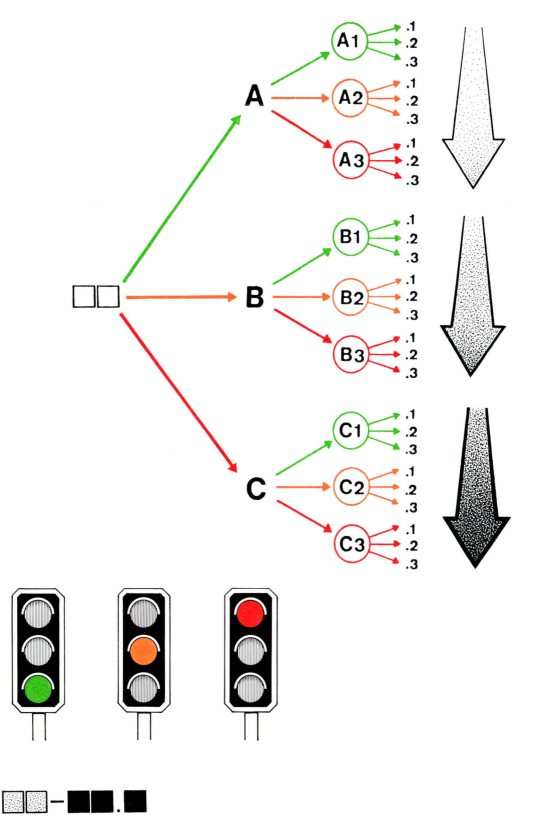

1.2   The Location

Each long bone or group of bones such as the spine is **designated by a number from 1 to 9**. The long bones humerus-**1**, radius/ulna-**2**, femur-**3** are further subdivided into 3 segments, denoted by the numbers 1, 2, 3; tibia/fibula-**4** is subdivided into 4 segments, denoted by the numbers 1, 2, 3, 4. This subdivision was necessary to permit the malleolar fractures to be represented as a separate segment. The 3 segments of the spine-**5** are cervical, thoracic, and lumbar. The pelvis-**6** is subdivided into 2 segments. The hand is designated by the number **7**, the foot by the number **8**. All the remaining bones are classified under the number **9**. In the first segment of 9 we find the patella (91.1), the clavicle (91.2), and the scapula (91.3). The second segment of 9 is reserved for mandibular fractures and the third for the facial bones and the skull. All illustrations in this book are drawn to represent the normal anatomical position as viewed from in front. All lateral views are represented with the anterior surface facing to the right.

1.3   Alpha-numeric Coding of the Diagnosis of a Fracture

Once the location has been determined, we combine it with the morphological characterization. This gives us the diagnosis. The codification is expressed in an alpha-numeric (letter, number) code to conform with computer practice. Each digit of the code has a specific significance. Together they convey the exact diagnosis and thus the severity of a particular fracture.

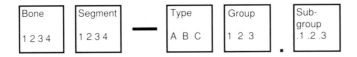

Within our system, the 9 principal bones with their 29 segments (pelvis 2 segments) when classified into the 3 fracture types which are divided into 3 groups and further subdivided into 3 subgroups give a potential classification of 783 fractures. If the additional qualification codes are added, more than 1500 fractures can be classified.

Fig. 2   **The bones and their segments. An overview of the whole skeleton**

1   Humerus and its 3 segments: proximal, diaphyseal, and distal
2   Radius/Ulna and its 3 segments: proximal, diaphyseal, and distal
3   Femur and its 3 segments: proximal, diaphyseal, and distal
4   Tibia/Fibula and its 4 segments: proximal, diaphyseal, distal, and malleolar
5   Spine and its 3 segments: cervical, thoracic, lumbar
6   Pelvis and its 2 segments: extra-articular and the acetabulum
7   Hand
8   Foot
9   Other bones: 91.1 Patella, 91.2 Clavicle, 91.3 Scapula, 92 Mandible, 93 Facial Bones and Skull

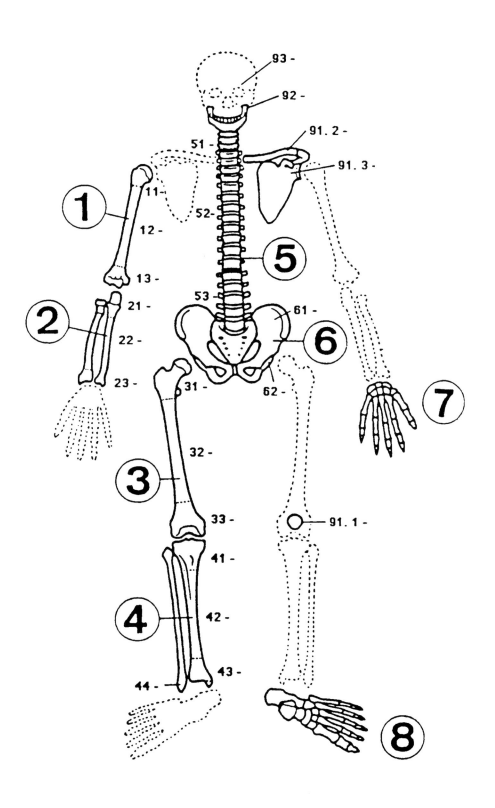

93 -

92 -

91. 2 -

91. 3 -

51 -

① 11-

12 -

52-

⑤

13 -

② 21 -

22 -

⑥ 61 -

23 -

31 - 62 -

32 -

③

33 -

91. 1 -

41 -

④ 42 -

43 -

44 -

⑦

⑧

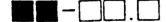

2. The Long Bones, General Comments

2.1   Coding of the Long Bones

The long bones are the humerus, the radius/ulna, the femur, and the tibia/fibula.

In the interest of clarity, all the bones have been drawn the same size.

> **Exception:** Page 11, the normal scale relationship of the bones has been observed in the illustration.

Fig. 3   **The long bones**

      1   Humerus
      2   Radius/Ulna
      3   Femur
      4   Tibia/Fibula
      The small squares: The blackened square indicates the portion of the alpha-numerical code being illustrated

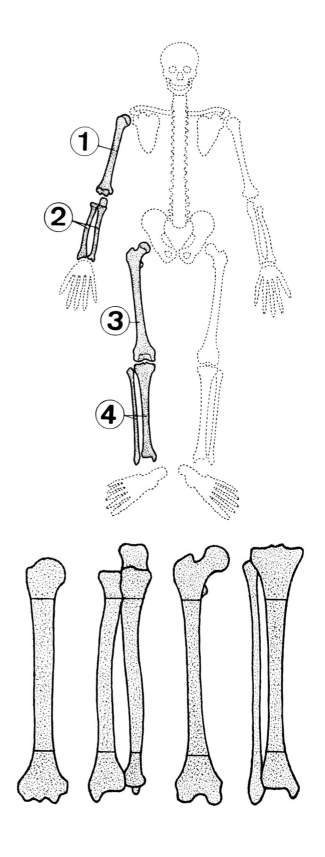

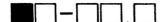

2.2 The Determination of the Segments of the Long Bones and of the Center of a Fracture

We define the diaphyseal segment of the long bones by defining the extent of the proximal and distal segments.

The **proximal** and **distal segments** comprise by definition the anatomical regions of the metaphysis and epiphysis. There are no standard radiological landmarks which separate the metaphysis and the diaphysis. An exception to this is the proximal femur. To aid in the definition of the diaphyseal-metaphyseal border, we have adopted the method of "squares" as proposed by Urs Heim. Although this system utilizes an arbitrary technique for defining the borders, it correlates well with the anatomical and clinical reality.

The system of "squares" is as follows: The proximal and distal segments of long bones are **defined by a square** whose sides are the same length as the widest part of the epiphysis in question.

> **Exceptions:**
> The **proximal femur** is defined as that portion proximal to a line which passes transversely through the inferior edge of the lesser trochanter.
> The **malleolar segment** is represented as segment **44-**. The malleoli are therefore not included in the square 43-

The **diaphyseal segments** are contained between the proximal and distal segments.

Before a fracture can be assigned to a segment one must first determine its **centre.** In a *simple fracture*, the **centre of the fracture** is obvious. In a *wedge fracture*, the centre is at the level of the broadest part of the wedge. In a *complex fracture*, the centre can be determined only after reduction.

Any **diaphyseal** fracture associated with a *displaced articular component* is considered as an *articular fracture*. If a fracture is associated only with an *undisplaced fissure* which reaches the joint, it is classified as a metaphyseal or diaphyseal fracture depending on its centre.

If one bone has **two completely separate fractures**, one of which is in the diaphysis and one in the proximal or distal segments (e.g. a femoral diaphysis and a femoral neck fracture), each fracture must be classified and coded separately.

Fig. 4   **The determination of the segments of long bones**

See also the text. The different squares are parallel to the long axis of the body and correspond to the end segments. The malleolar segment (44-) is not represented here as it cannot be compared with the other end segments

10

11 –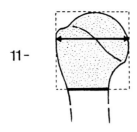

31 –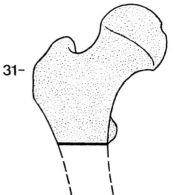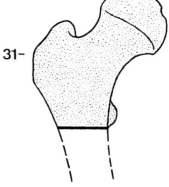

12 –

32 –

13 –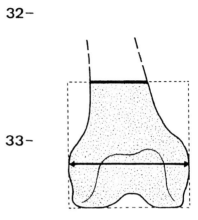

33 –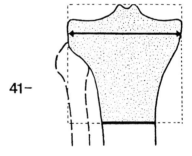

21 –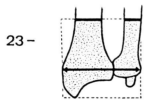

41 –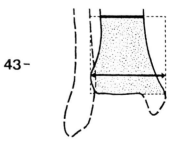

22 –

42 –

23 –

43 –

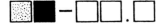 ▨■ – □□.□

11

2.3 The Classification of Diaphyseal Fractures

In general, the classification of diaphyseal fractures is not particularly difficult since these fractures are quite similar.

As indicated in the section on general principles of classification (p. 6), the first step is to assign the fracture to one of the three types: **A, B,** or **C.** The second step is to assign the fracture to one of the three groups. The third step is to assign the fracture to one of the three subgroups.

Fig. 5   The scheme of the **morphological characterization** of the fractures of the diaphyseal segment

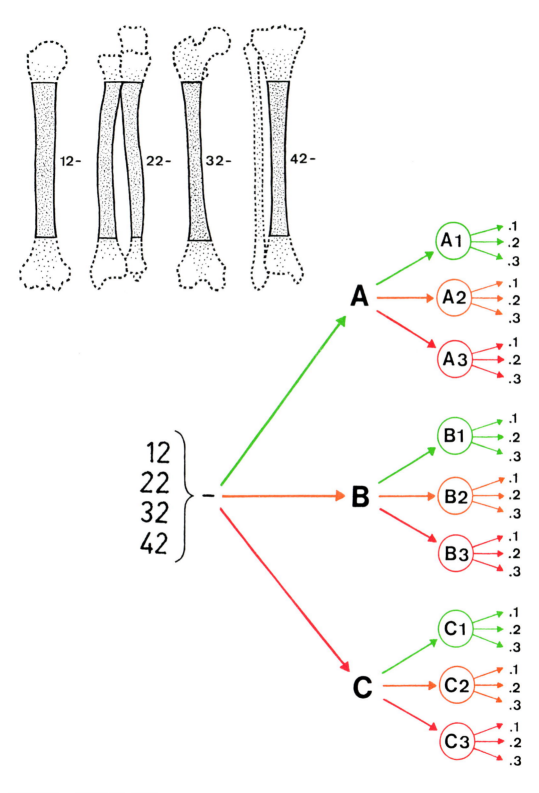

12–
22–
32–
42–

12
22
32
42

A
A1 .1 .2 .3
A2 .1 .2 .3
A3 .1 .2 .3

B
B1 .1 .2 .3
B2 .1 .2 .3
B3 .1 .2 .3

C
C1 .1 .2 .3
C2 .1 .2 .3
C3 .1 .2 .3

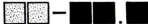

2.3.1   The Diaphyseal Fracture Types

The fractures of the diaphyseal segment of long bones are divided into three types: **A, B,** and **C.**
The order of the letters indicates increasing severity. The meaning of the types is identical for all
fractures of the diaphyseal segment of long bones.

Fractures of long bones are either *simple* or *multifragmentary*:

Type A represents *simple fractures* with two fragments. These are characterized by a single
cortical disruption of at least 90% of the circumference of the bone.

Types B and C represent the two types of *multifragmentary fractures*:

Type B represents fractures with a wedge fragment. We refer to these as *wedge fractures.*
These are characterized by the fact that after reduction there is always some contact between the
main fragments and that reduction of the main fracture line usually restores the normal length and
alignment of the bone.

Type C represents the *complex fractures*. In these after reduction there is no contact between
the main fragments.

> **Please note:** Types **B** and **C** comprise fractures with more than two fragments. These
> can therefore be referred to as **multifragmentary fractures** in distinction to the **simple
> fractures** Type A.

Fig. 6   **The diaphyseal fracture types**

  A   Simple fracture
  B   Wedge fracture
  C   Complex fracture

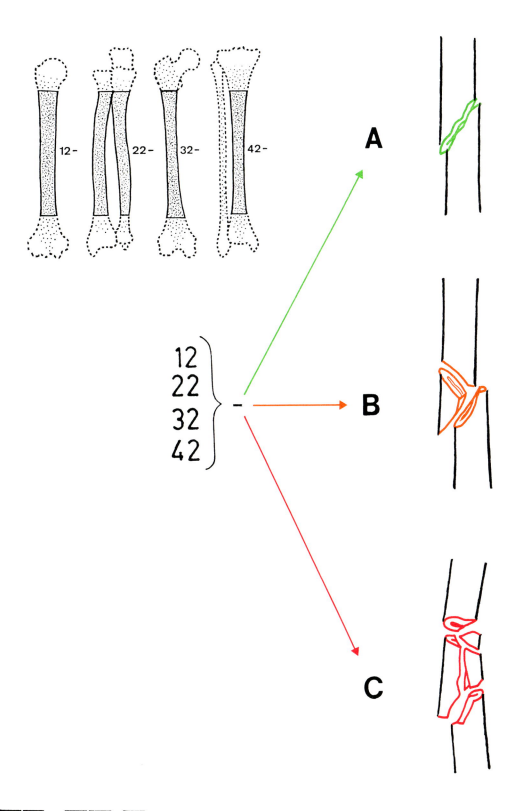

12
22
32
42

A

B

C

15

2.3.2 The Groups of the Diaphyseal Fractures of the Humerus, Femur, and Tibia/Fibula

Each of the fracture Types **A**, **B**, and **C** of the diaphysis of the humerus, femur, and tibia/fibula are further subdivided into three groups denoted by the numbers **1, 2, 3.** In the classification the nine groups are coded by combining the letter for the fracture type with the number representing its subdivision.

All spiral fractures, the result of torsion, are found in the groups A1, B1, and C1, that is the first subdivision of the respective types. All the other fracture shapes such as the wedge fractures and the complex fractures, which are the result of bending, are assigned to the remaining groups.

Type A (simple fractures) is divided into three groups of increasing severity as follows: **A1 =** *simple fracture, spiral*; **A2** = *simple fracture, oblique*; **A3** = *simple fracture, transverse.* Thus, the Type A fractures give rise to 3 fracture Groups: A1, A2, and A3. The Groups A2 and A3 are distinguished from one another by the angle which the fracture line subtends with a perpendicular to the long axis of the bone. If the angle is equal to or greater than 30 degrees, the fracture is considered as oblique (A2); if it is less than 30 degrees, transverse (A3).

Type B fractures (wedge fractures) are subdivided into 3 groups of increasing severity as follows: **B1** = *spiral wedge*, **B2** = *bending wedge*, and **B3** = *fragmented wedge.* B 1 is the result of torsion. B2 and B3 are the result of bending. B3 arises when the intermediate wedge is fragmented by bending forces. In the B fractures, after reduction, there is always some contact between the main fragments.

Type C fractures (complex fractures) are fractures with *multiple wedge fragments or with segmentation.* In these after reduction there is no contact between the main fragments. As all spiral fractures are classified into the first group of the fracture types, the classification is as follows: **C1** = *complex fracture, spiral*; **C2** = *complex fracture, segmental*; and **C3** = *complex fracture, irregular.*

Fig. 7   **The groups of the diaphyseal fractures of the Humerus, Femur, and Tibia/Fibula**

A1   Simple fracture, spiral
A2   Simple fracture, oblique ($\geq 30°$)
A3   Simple fracture, transverse ($< 30°$)

B1   Wedge fracture, spiral wedge
B2   Wedge fracture, bending wedge
B3   Wedge fracture, fragmented wedge

C1   Complex fracture, spiral
C2   Complex fracture, segmental
C3   Complex fracture, irregular

16

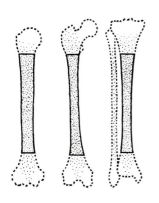

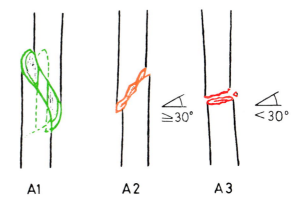

A1   A2   A3

$\geqq 30°$ $< 30°$

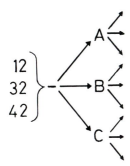

12
32 }
42

A
B
C

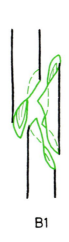 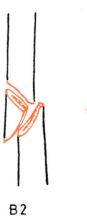 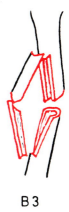

B1   B2   B3

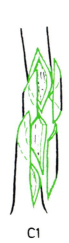 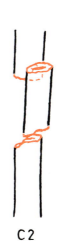 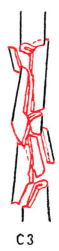

C1   C2   C3

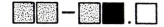

17

2.3.3 The Groups of the Diaphyseal Fractures of the Radius/Ulna

The presence of two bones in the forearm has forced a modification of the classification system. Because spiral fractures of these two bones are rare (p. 21), the forearm fractures are classified according to the involvement of one or both bones. Each of the three fracture types of the forearm is subdivided into three groups according to the severity of the fracture and according to the specific bone involved. Fractures of the ulna occupy the first level of severity, those of the radius the second, and both bone fractures of equal complexity the third or highest level of severity. It follows thus that complex fractures C1 relate to the ulna and C2 to the radius, while C3 denotes a complex fracture of both bones.

In the Type **A**, we have three groups: A1 = simple fracture of the ulna; A2 = simple fracture of the radius; A3 = simple fracture of both bones.

In the Type **B** (wedge fractures), we have three groups: B1 = wedge fracture of the ulna, radius intact; B2 = wedge fracture of the radius, ulna intact; B3 = wedge fracture of one bone, with a simple or wedge fracture of the other.

In subdividing the Type **C**, we are governed by the site of the complex fracture. Thus, C1 = complex fracture of the ulna with the radius being either intact or having a simple or wedge fracture; C2 = complex fracture of the radius with the ulna being intact or having either a simple or a wedge fracture; and C3 = complex fracture of both bones.

> **Please note:** In order to classify further the Monteggia and Galeazzi fractures we must resort to the subgroups (see pp. 100-105).

Fig. 8   **The groups of the diaphyseal fractures of the Radius/Ulna**

A1	Simple fracture of the ulna, radius intact
A2	Simple fracture of the radius, ulna intact
A3	Simple fracture of both bones
B1	Wedge fracture of the ulna, radius intact
B2	Wedge fracture of the radius, ulna intact
B3	Wedge fracture of one bone, simple or wedge fracture of the other
C1	Complex fracture of the ulna
C2	Complex fracture of the radius
C3	Complex fracture of both bones

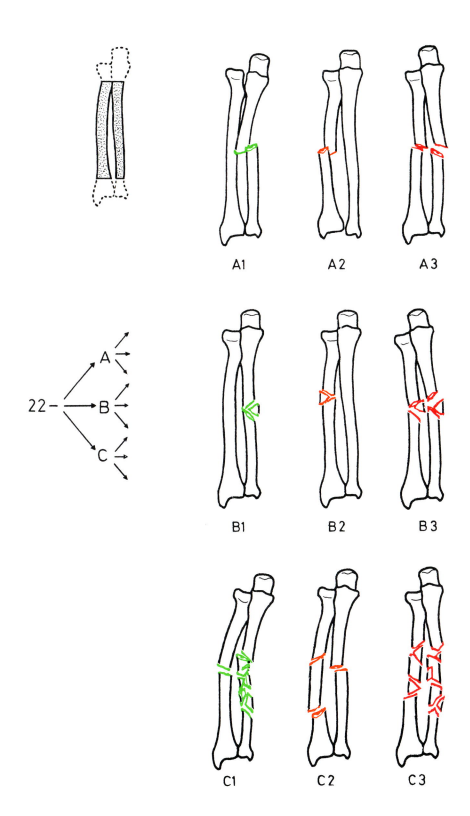

A1 A2 A3

22 → A
    → B
    → C

B1 B2 B3

C1 C2 C3

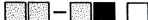

19

2.3.4 A Comparative Analysis of 2700 Surgically Treated Diaphyseal Fractures (Fig. 9)

The table presents the relative incidence of the groups of diaphyseal fractures. Of particular note is the rarity of spiral fractures of the radius and ulna (less than 1%). For this reason, the spiral fractures of the radius and ulna are grouped with the bending fractures and are classed as either simple or as wedge fractures.

Each **fracture type** occurs with similar frequency in the four bones: Type **A** = 61% in the humerus, 65% in the radius/ulna, 53% in the femur, and 45% in the tibia/fibula; Type **B** = 32% in the humerus, 29% in the radius/ulna, 34% in the femur, and 46% in the tibia/fibula; Type **C** = 7% in the humerus, 6% in the radius/ulna, 13% in the femur, and 9% in the tibia/fibula.

The **groups** are similar in the humerus, femur and tibia/fibula. For example, spiral fractures represent 27% of fractures in the humerus, 23% of fractures in the femur, and 25% of the tibial fractures.

It is interesting to note that the complex spiral fractures comprise only 3% of the fractures of the humerus, 4% of the fractures of the femur, and 1% of the fractures of the tibia/fibula. Segmental fractures are rare in the humerus (1%), but show an increasing incidence in the femur and tibia/fibula (4% and 6% respectively). Complex irregular fractures comprise 3% of the diaphyseal fractures of the humerus, 5% of the diaphyseal fractures of the femur, and 2% of the tibial diaphyseal fractures.

Among the fracture types of radius/ulna we see an incidence of Type A (simple) as follows: 18% simple fractures of the ulna, 21% simple fractures of the radius, and 26% simple fractures of both bones.
The incidence of Type B (wedge fractures) is as follows: 7% wedge fractures of the ulna, 8% of the radius, and 14% of both bones.
The incidence of Type C (complex fractures) is as follows: 2% of the ulna, 2% of the radius, and 2% of both bones.

			A	**B**	**C**	
12-	N =	200 :	61 %	32 %	7 %	= 100 %
22-	N =	500 :	65 %	29 %	6 %	= 100 %
32-	N =	1000 :	53 %	34 %	13 %	= 100 %
42-	N =	1000 :	45 %	46 %	9 %	= 100 %

A: **12-A** = 61%, **22-A** = 65%, **32-A** = 53%, **42-A** = 45%

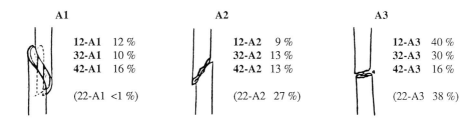

	A1		A2		A3
12-A1	12 %	**12-A2**	9 %	**12-A3**	40 %
32-A1	10 %	**32-A2**	13 %	**32-A3**	30 %
42-A1	16 %	**42-A2**	13 %	**42-A3**	16 %
(22-A1 <1 %)		(22-A2 27 %)		(22-A3 38 %)	

B: **12-B** = 32%, **22-B** = 29%, **32-B** = 34%, **42-B** = 46%

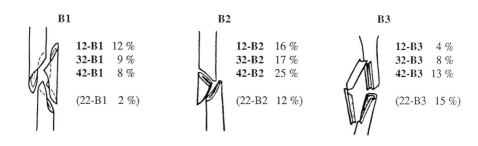

	B1		B2		B3
12-B1	12 %	**12-B2**	16 %	**12-B3**	4 %
32-B1	9 %	**32-B2**	17 %	**32-B3**	8 %
42-B1	8 %	**42-B2**	25 %	**42-B3**	13 %
(22-B1 2 %)		(22-B2 12 %)		(22-B3 15 %)	

C: **12-C** = 7%, **22-C** = 6%, **32-C** = 13%, **42-C** = 9%

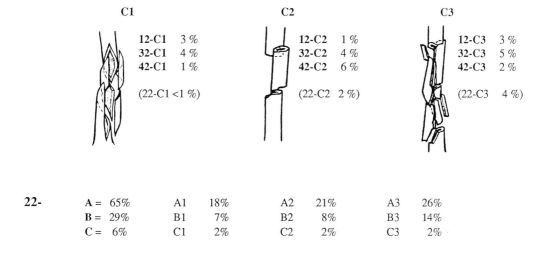

	C1		C2		C3
12-C1	3 %	**12-C2**	1 %	**12-C3**	3 %
32-C1	4 %	**32-C2**	4 %	**32-C3**	5 %
42-C1	1 %	**42-C2**	6 %	**42-C3**	2 %
(22-C1 <1 %)		(22-C2 2 %)		(22-C3 4 %)	

22-							
	A = 65%	A1	18%	A2	21%	A3	26%
	B = 29%	B1	7%	B2	8%	B3	14%
	C = 6%	C1	2%	C2	2%	C3	2%

2.3.5 The Subgroups .1, .2, and .3 of the Diaphyseal Groups A1, A2, A3, and B1, B2, B3

The diaphyseal groups are further subdivided into three subgroups: .1, .2, .3. The distinguishing features of the subgroups differ from bone to bone.

The subgroups for the groups **A** and **B** are similar for the **humerus** and the **femur**. They indicate the **level of the fracture**. Thus, .1 stands for **proximal zone**, .2 for **middle zone**, and .3 for **distal zone**.

> **Please note:**
> Subtrochanteric fractures of the femur involve the portion of the shaft which extends from a transverse line drawn through the inferior border of the lesser trochanter to a point 3 cm distal to it. The subtrochanteric fractures are therefore classified within a different segment than the intertrochanteric fractures which are classified with the proximal segment of the femur.
> The proximal diaphysis of the humerus is the zone of the **proximal diaphyseal flare**. In both the femur and humerus, the zone is proportionately quite short.
> By definition, the middle diaphysis applies to the **zone with a uniform medullary canal** diameter.
> The distal diaphysis is the zone of the **distal diaphyseal flare** which is much longer in the femur than in the humerus.

In fractures of the **tibia/fibula** the subgroups reflect the presence or absence of a fibular fracture as well as its level. Thus: .1 = fibula intact, .2 = fibula fractured at another level than that in the tibia, and .3 = fibula fractured at the same level as the tibia.

> **Please note:** The intact fibula splints and stabilizes the fractured tibia. It does not contribute to delayed union as long as the fracture is properly treated and closely followed. If the fracture of the fibula is at a level remote from the fracture of the tibia, the tibia is less stable, but the fibula is still able to splint the tibia through the fibres of the interosseous membrane. In contrast, fractures of the fibula and tibia at the same level are very unstable.

The classification of **radius/ulna fractures** differs in that the group denotes the bone involved (ulna, radius, or ulna and radius) (see pages 98 to 105).

Fig. 10 **The subgroups of the diaphyseal groups A1, A2, A3, and B1, B2, and B3**

Humerus and Femur	.1	proximal zone (= subtrochanteric in the femur)
	.2	middle zone
	.3	distal zone
Tibia/Fibula	.1	fibula intact
	.2	fibula fractured at an other level
	.3	fibula fractured at the same level
Radius/Ulna		please see pages 100-103

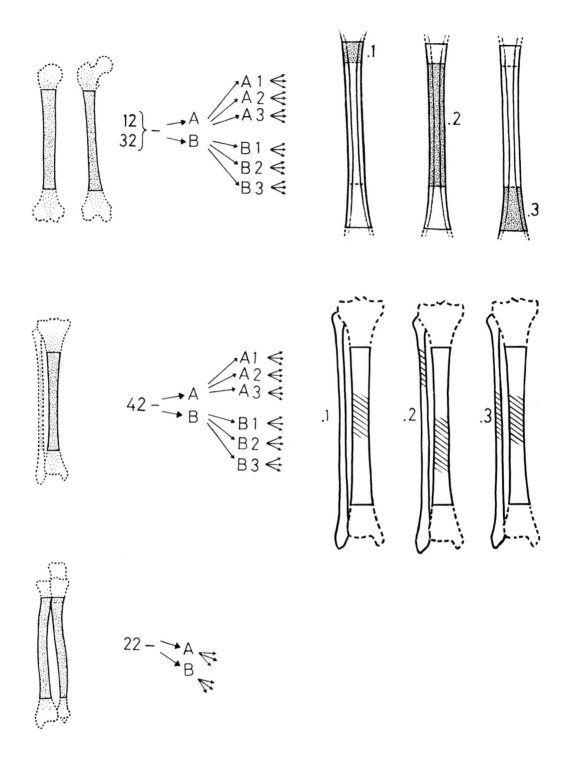

23

2.3.6 The Subgroups .1, .2, and .3 of the Diaphyseal Groups C1, C2, C3

These subgroups are identical in the complex fractures of the humerus, femur and tibia. In fractures of the forearm the system differs because here either one or both bones can be involved.

The Groups **C1** (the complex spiral fractures) are subdivided into subgroups on the basis of the number of intermediate fracture fragments.

The Groups **C2** (the complex segmental fractures) are differentiated into subgroups according to the presence of additional wedge fragments or an additional segmental level. Complex segmental fractures in which the intermediate fragment is split longitudinally are classified with the C3 group as C3.1.

The Groups **C3** (the complex irregular fractures) are differentiated into subgroups according to the number of the intermediate fragments and the extension of the fracture. The Subgroups C3.2 and C3.3 are more aptly referred to as *shattered fractures* as the number of the intermediate fragments is difficult to determine.

If one cannot determine the subgroup, then it is coded as **Subgroup .4** and the fracture pattern is described verbally.

Fig. 11   **The subgroups of the diaphyseal groups C1, C2, and C3 for the Humerus, Femur and the Tibia/Fibula**

C1 Complex fracture, spiral
.1   with two intermediate fragments
.2   with three intermediate fragments
.3   with more than three intermediate fragments

C2 Complex fracture, segmental
.1   with an intermediate segmental fragment
.2   with an intermediate segmental and additional wedge fragment(s)
.3   with two intermediate segmental fragments

C3 Complex fracture, irregular
.1   with 2-3 intermediate fragments
.2   with limited shattering (< 5 cm)
.3   with extensive shattering (≥ 5 cm)

Radius/Ulna: see pages 104 and 105

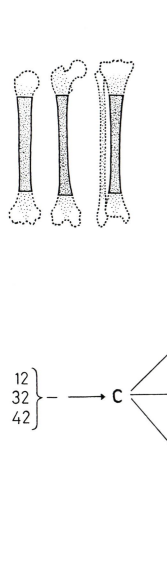

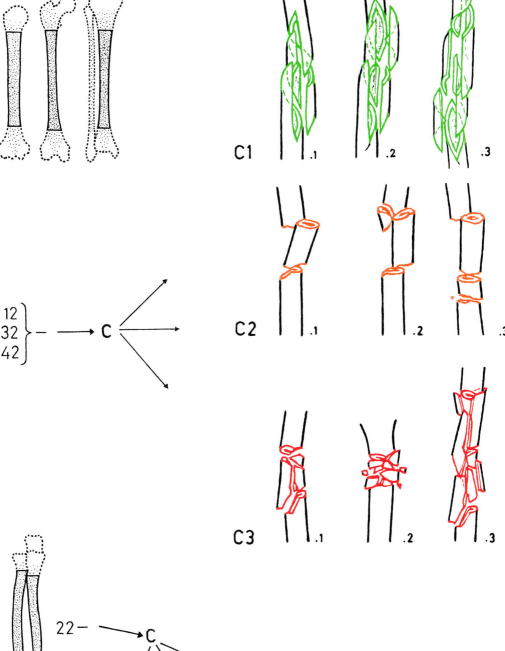

$$\left.\begin{matrix} 12 \\ 32 \\ 42 \end{matrix}\right\} - \longrightarrow C$$

C1 .1 .2 .3

C2 .1 .2 .3

C3 .1 .2 .3

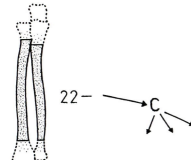

$$22 - \longrightarrow C$$

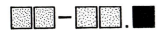

2.3.7   The Qualifications for the Diaphyseal Subgroups

The qualifications afford an extra level of precision in defining the subgroups. Previously the surgeon had to describe in **long hand** the various qualifications of the fracture. In the new system we have evolved, the surgeon simply identifies the appropriate qualification by a number from 1 to 9 and enters this number in parentheses directly following the number denoting the subgroup. In the qualifications numbered from 1 to 6, the first code number listed in parentheses conveys additional information about the fracture location and extent and the second adds more descriptive information. Three additional qualifications remain: *7)* represents a *partial amputation, 8)* a *total amputation* and *9)* a *loss of bony substance.*

We shall use here as an example the subgroups of the Group **C2**, which we have described on the preceding page. The code for the qualifications are printed in italics and as a rule are not depicted diagramatically.

Whenever one or more qualifications are to be added to the subgroups, they are placed in parentheses (see small squares).

Fig. 12   **Example: Qualifications for the diaphyseal subgroups of C2**

C2.1   Complex fracture, with an intermediate segmental fragment
      1) pure diaphyseal
      2) proximal diaphysio-metaphyseal
      3) distal diaphysio-metaphyseal
      4) oblique lines
      5) transverse and oblique lines

C2.2   Complex fracture with an intermediate segmental and additional wedge fragment(s)
      1) pure diaphyseal
      2) proximal diaphysio-metaphyseal
      3) distal diaphysio-metaphyseal
      4) distal wedge
      5) two wedges, proximal and distal

C2.3   Complex fracture, with two intermediate segmental fragments
      1) pure diaphyseal
      2) proximal diaphysio-metaphyseal
      3) distal diaphysio-metaphyseal

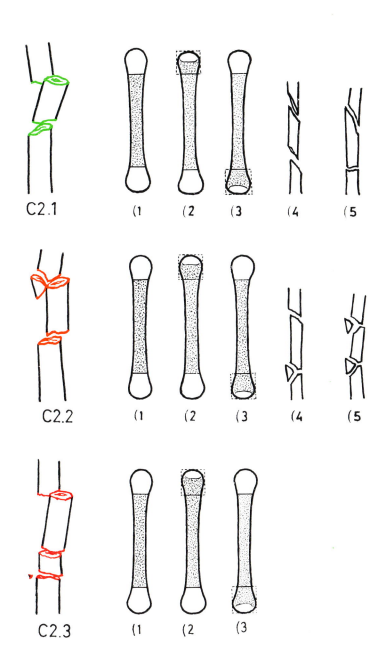

C2.1   (1   (2   (3   (4   (5

C2.2   (1   (2   (3   (4   (5

C2.3   (1   (2   (3

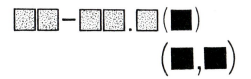

2.4   The Classification of Fractures of the Proximal and Distal Segments

In order to classify fractures of the proximal and distal segments of the long bones, we use the same system of fracture types, groups, and subgroups. We also use the criteria of severity in differentiating between them and in arranging them in ascending order.

The classification system does not apply as uniformly in the 4 proximal and 5 distal segments as it does in diaphyseal fractures.

The architecture and shape of the various proximal and distal segments is quite varied as are the mechanisms of injury (flexion, avulsion, shearing, and axial and lateral compression).

The humeral and femoral heads, because of their direct articulation with the trunk, have not only a much greater range of motion, but their anatomy also differs from the other more peripheral joints. Also the anatomical features of the malleolar segment are unique.

When we exclude these three peculiar segments, the proximal humerus, the proximal femur, and the malleolar segment, we are left with 6 segments which can be classified systematically. These are: 13- = the distal humerus, 21- = the proximal radius/ulna, 23- = the distal radius/ulna, 33- = the distal femur, 41- = the proximal tibia/fibula, and 43- = the distal tibia/fibula.

Fig. 13   **The scheme of the morphological characterization of the fractures of the proximal and distal segments**

    The segments 13- and 33-, 21- and 41- , and 23- and 43- have identical fracture types
    The segments 11- and 31- have similar fracture types
    The malleolar segment 44- is unique

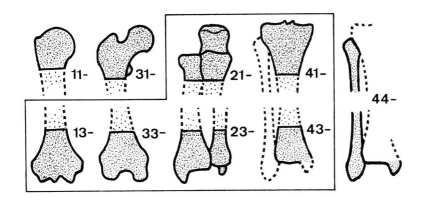

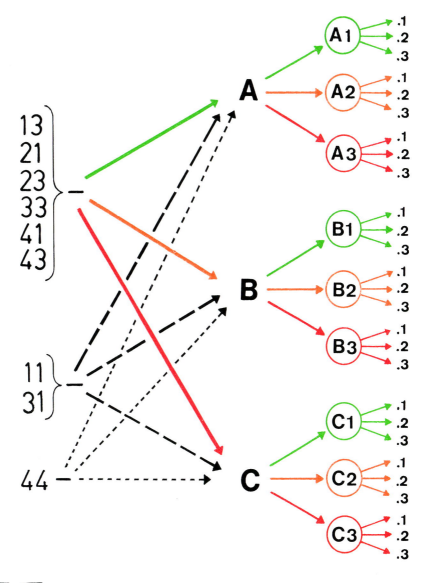

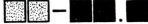

2.4.1   The Fracture Types of Segments 13- and 33-, 21- and 41-, 23- and 43-

As in fractures of the diaphyseal segments, the fractures of the proximal and distal segments are divided into three fracture types. With the exception of the proximal humerus and proximal femur, **Type A** generally indicates extra-articular fractures, **Type B** partial articular fractures, and **Type C** complete articular fractures. Because of the morphological similarities between the humerus and femur and as well as between the radius/ulna and tibia/fibula, we have grouped these regions together in figure 14 with the analagous segments side by side.

Type A represents all *extra-articular fractures.* The fracture line may be metaphyseal or epiphyseal, but it always spares the articular surface although it may be intracapsular.

Type B represents *partial articular fractures.* In these, the fracture involves part of the articular surface while the remainder of the joint remains intact and is solidly connected to the supporting metaphysis and diaphysis. In classifying fractures of the proximal radius and ulna the two bones are considered as a single functional unit. Thus, a partial articular fracture of the proximal radius/ulna involves an articular fracture of either the radius or the ulna while the other bone is either spared or has an extra-articular fracture.

Type C represents *complete articular fractures.* These are characterized by a disruption of the articular surface and its complete separation from the diaphysis.

In the accompanying illustration the solid white areas indicate an intact articular surface and represent Type A fractures whereas the checkered pattern represents the Type C fracture. The methaphysis is depicted in horizontal stripes for both fracture types. The severity of the extra-articular component of the Type C fracture will determine whether it falls into the first or the second group, that is C1 or C2.

Because of their unique anatomy, the proximal humerus, the proximal femur, and the malleolar segments are dealt with separately on the following pages.

Fig. 14   **The fracture types of the segments 13- and 33-, 21- and 41-, 23- and 43-.**

    A   Extra-articular fracture
    B   Partial articular fracture
    C   Complete articular fracture

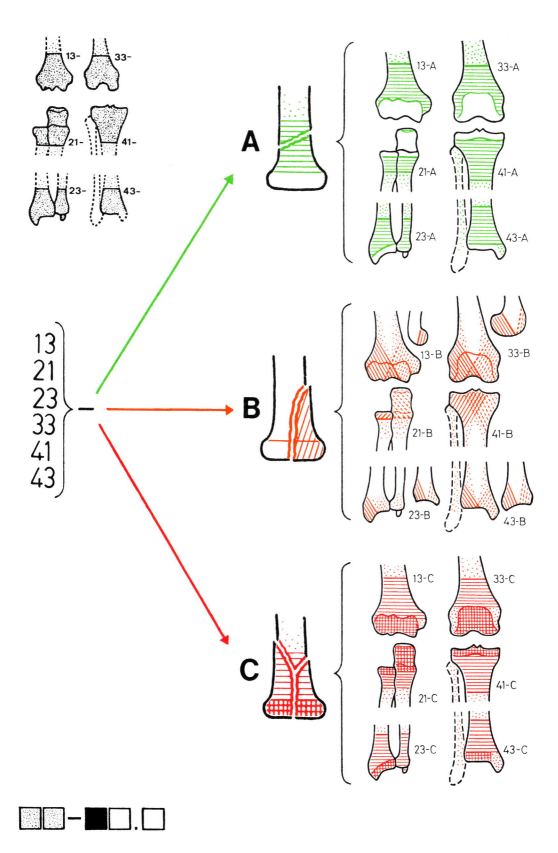

2.4.2   The Fracture Types for the Segments 11- and 31-

Type A represents the *simple extra-articular* fractures of the proximal humerus which involve one tuberosity or the metaphysis (unifocal); it represents in the proximal femur fractures involving the **intertrochanteric area.**

Type B for the proximal humerus represents *extra-articular* fractures which involve one tuberosity and the metaphysis (bifocal); it represents in the proximal femur fractures of the **neck.**

Type C for the proximal humerus represents *articular* fractures which involve the **anatomical neck** of the humerus; it represents for the proximal femur the fractures of the **head.**

> **Please note:** The **groups** are represented on pp. 46-49

2.4.3   The Fracture Types for the Segment 44-

These fracture types are distinguished from one another by the level of the accompanying fibular fracture and the condition of the syndesmotic ligaments. Thus, the fracture Type **A** represents fibular fractures below the syndesmosis (infrasyndesmotic), Type **B** represents fibular fractures at the level of the syndesmosis (transsyndesmotic), and Type **C** represents fibular fractures above the syndesmosis (suprasyndesmotic).

Fig. 15   **The fracture types for the segments 11-, 31-, and 44-**

11-   **Humerus proximal**
A   Extra-articular unifocal fracture
B   Extra-articular bifocal fracture
C   Articular fracture

31-   **Femur proximal**
A   Trochanteric area fracture
B   Neck fracture
C   Head fracture

44-   **Malleolar segment**
A   Infrasyndesmotic lesion
B   Transsyndesmotic fibula fracture
C   Suprasyndesmotic lesion

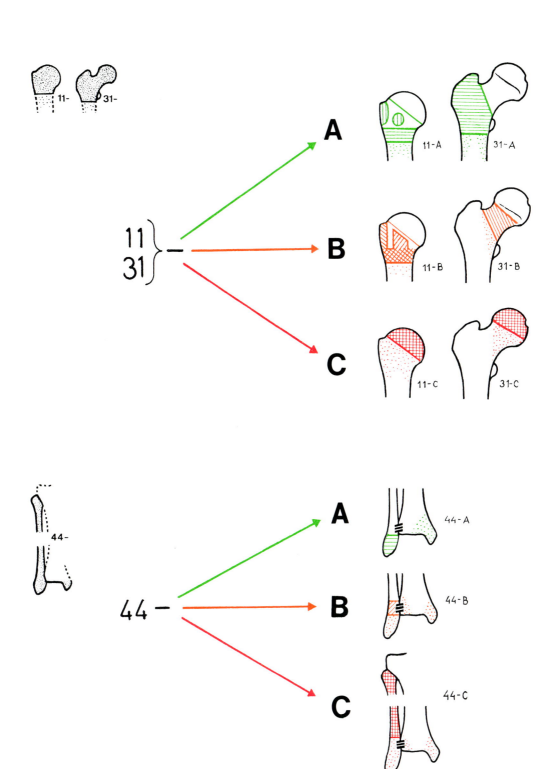

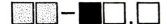

2.4.4   The Groups A1, A2, A3 of the Segments 13-, 21- and 23-, 33-, 41- and 43-

The **Groups A1, A2, A3** represent the *extra-articular* fractures. They are either avulsions of **tendinous** or ligamentous insertion from apophyses, or more often they are either simple metaphyseal fractures or multifragmentary metaphyseal fractures with (a) wedge fragment(s). *Impacted fractures* are usually stable simple fractures of the metaphysis or epiphysis in which the cortex of one fragment is **driven into** the cancellous bone of **the other.** A pure *compression* fracture can occur in the metaphysis of the distal radius/tibia. In the adult, *multifragmentary* cortical fractures are usually associated with a certain degree of compression

In the **distal humerus,** the epicondylar avulsions are classified as A1, the simple extra-articular metaphyseal fractures as A2, and the multifragmentary extra-articular metaphyseal fractures as A3.

In the **proximal radius/ulna,** A1 represents isolated simple fractures of the ulna, A2 isolated simple fractures of the radius, and A3 simple fractures of both the radius and ulna.

In the **distal radius/ulna,** A1 represents isolated extra-articular fractures of the ulna, A2 isolated simple extra-articular fractures of the radius, and A3 represents multifragmentary extra-articular fractures of the distal radius with varying degrees of compression.

Fig. 16   **The groups A1, A2, A3 of the upper extremity (segments 13-, 21-, 23-)**

13-   Humerus distal
   A1   Extra-articular fracture, apophyseal avulsion
   A2   Extra-articular fracture, metaphyseal simple
   A3   Extra-articular fracture, metaphyseal multifragmentary

21-   Radius/Ulna proximal
   A1   Extra-articular fracture, of the ulna, radius intact
   A2   Extra-articular fracture, of the radius, ulna intact
   A3   Extra-articular fracture, of both bones

23-   Radius/Ulna distal
   A1   Extra-articular fracture, of the ulna, radius intact
   A2   Extra-articular fracture, of the radius, simple and impacted
   A3   Extra-articular fracture, of the radius, multifragmentary

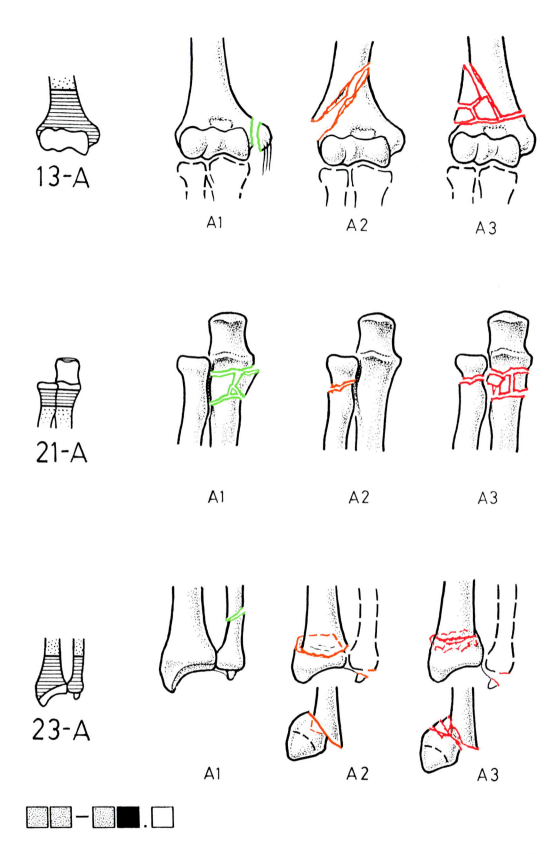

13-A

A1   A2   A3

21-A

A1   A2   A3

23-A

A1   A2   A3

In the **distal femur**, group **A1** represents the extra-articular (supracondylar) *simple* fractures, **A2** the metaphyseal wedge fractures, and **A3** the metaphyseal complex fractures.

In the **proximal tibia/fibula**, **A1** represents the avulsion fractures, **A2** the metaphyseal simple fractures, and **A3** the metaphyseal multifragmentary fractures.

In the **distal tibia/fibula**, **A1** represents the metaphyseal simple fractures, **A2** the metaphyseal fractures with a wedge fragment, and **A3** the metaphyseal complex fractures.

Please note:
1) The terminology for the 41-A and the 43-A fractures has been unified under the term **"metaphyseal"** which has replaced **"supramalleolar"** for the distal tibia and the term **"supracondylar"** for fractures type 13-A and 33-A.
2) In the case of multifragmentary diaphyseal fractures the result of great compressive forces, the cortex is shattered (see 23-A3).

Exception: As an exception to the rule that only extra-articular fractures are classified as Type A, we have classified the fractures of the **intercondylar tibial eminence** as A despite the fact that they usually involve a small portion of the adjacent articular cartilage. These are classified as A1 lesions.

Fig. 17   **The groups A1, A2, A3 of segments 33-, 41- and 43-** (lower extremity)

33-   Femur distal
    A1   Extra-articular fracture, simple
    A2   Extra-articular fracture, metaphyseal wedge
    A3   Extra-articular fracture, metaphyseal complex

41-   Tibia/Fibula proximal
    A1   Extra-articular fracture, avulsion
    A2   Extra-articular fracture, metaphyseal simple
    A3   Extra-articular fracture, metaphyseal multifragmentary

43-   Tibia/Fibula distal
    A1   Extra-articular fracture, metaphyseal simple
    A2   Extra-articular fracture, metaphyseal wedge
    A3   Extra-articular fracture, metaphyseal complex

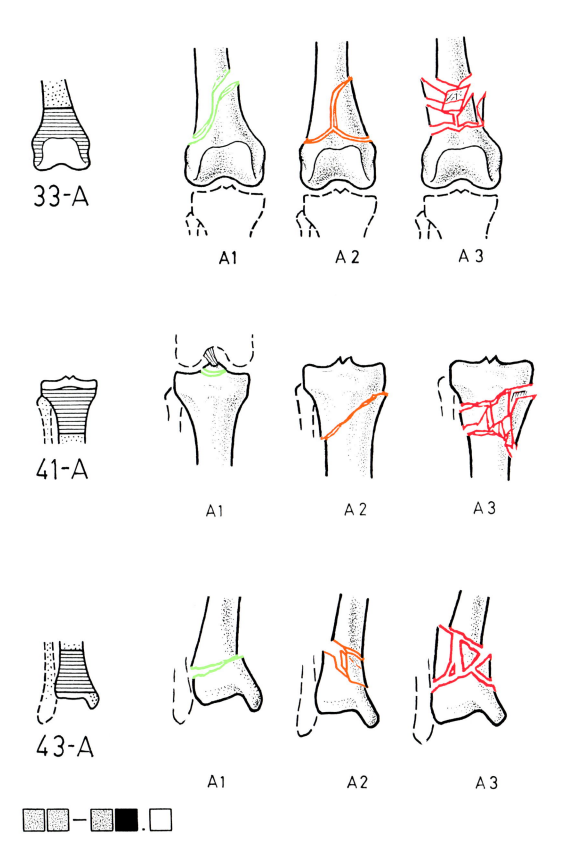

33-A

A1 A2 A3

41-A

A1 A2 A3

43-A

A1 A2 A3

2.4.5 The Groups B1, B2, B3 of the Segments 13- ,21- ,23- ,33- ,41-, and 43-

The fracture Type **B** represents *partial articular fractures* in which part of the joint retains its continuity with the diaphysis.

In the **distal humerus**, the partial articular fractures, which involve the lateral part of the joint are classified as B1, those involving the medial part as B2, and those which are in the frontal plane as B3.

In the **proximal radius/ulna**, partial articular fractures are classified as follows: The Group B1 represents the isolated articular fractures of the ulna (olecranon), B2 the isolated articular fractures of the radius (radial head), and B3 the articular fractures of one of the two bones associated with an extra-articular fracture of the other.

In the **distal radius/ulna**, B1 are the articular fractures of the radius in the sagittal plane, B2 the partial articular dorsal rim fractures (Barton), and B3 the volar articular rim fractures (reverse Barton, Goyrand-Smith II).

Fig. 18   **The groups B1, B2, B3 of segments 13-, 21-, and 23-**

13- Humerus distal
B1   Partial articular fracture, lateral sagittal
B2   Partial articular fracture, medial sagittal
B3   Partial articular fracture, frontal

21- Radius/Ulna proximal
B1   Articular fracture, of the ulna, radius intact
B2   Articular fracture, of the radius, ulna intact
B3   Articular fracture, of the one bone, extra-articular fracture of the other

23- Radius/Ulna distal
B1   Partial articular fracture, of the radius, sagittal
B2   Partial articular fracture, of the radius, dorsal rim (Barton)
B3   Partial articular fracture, of the radius, volar rim (reverse Barton, Goyrand-Smith II)

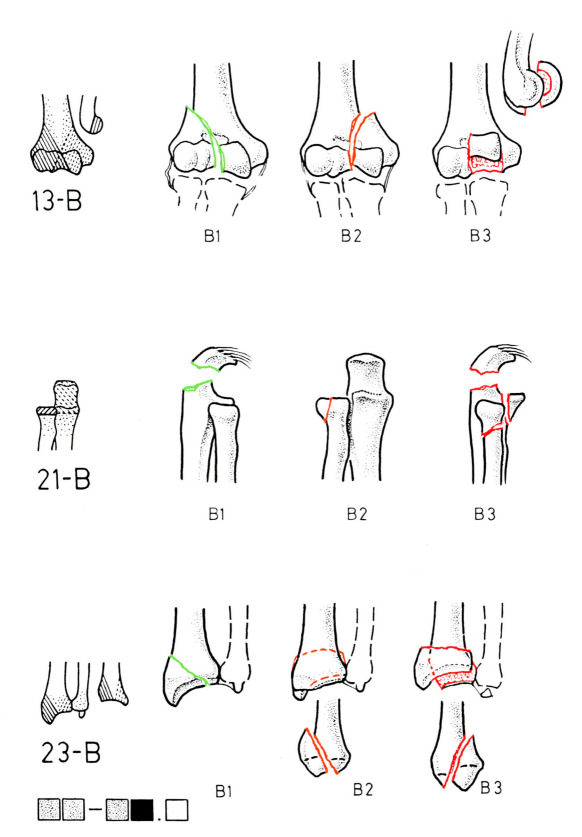

13-B

B1   B2   B3

21-B

B1   B2   B3

23-B

B1   B2   B3

The Long Bones, General Comments (Cont.)

In the **distal femur** the Group B1 represents the unicondylar fractures of the lateral condyle, B2 the unicondylar fractures of the medial condyle, and B3 the condylar fractures in the frontal plane (Hoffa).

In the **proximal tibia/fibula,** the Group B1 represents a pure split fracture, B2 the pure depression, and B3 the split with depression.

In the **distal tibia/fibula,** the Group B1 represents a pure split, B2 a split with a depression, and B3 a depression with fragmentation and dissociation of the articular fragments which are referred to as partial articular fracture, multifragmentary depressed.

Fig. 19   **The groups B1, B2, B3 of segments 33-, 41- and 43-**

33- Femur distal
B1   Partial articular fracture, lateral condyle, sagittal
B2   Partial articular fracture, medial condyle, sagittal
B3   Partial articular fracture, frontal

41- Tibia/Fibula proximal
B1   Partial articular fracture, pure split
B2   Partial articular fracture, pure depression
B3   Partial articular fracture, split-depression

43- Tibia/Fibula distal
B1   Partial articular fracture, pure split
B2   Partial articular fracture, split-depression
B3   Partial articular fracture, multifragmentary depression

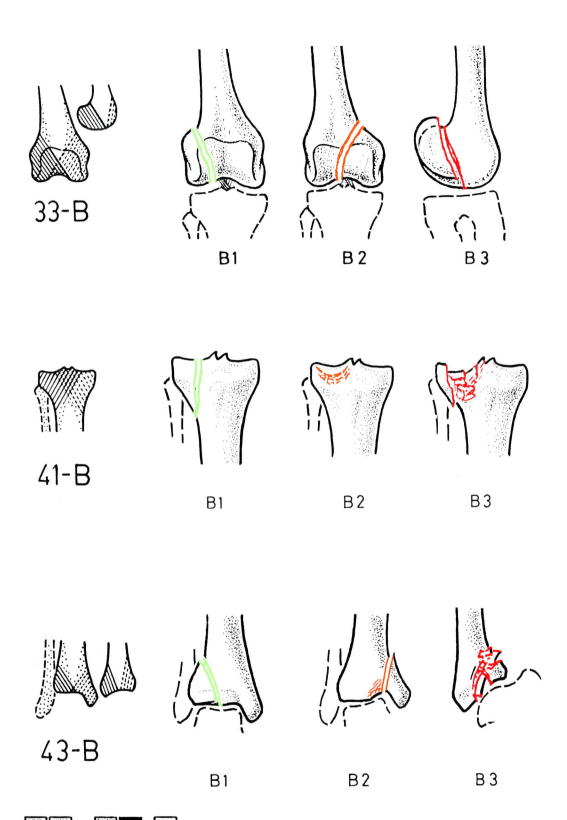

33-B

B1   B2   B3

41-B

B1   B2   B3

43-B

B1   B2   B3

2.4.6 The Groups C1, C2, C3 of the Segments 13-, 21- and 23-, 33-, 41- and 43-

The fracture Type C represents *complete articular fractures* (see p. 30) in which the articular surface is completely separated from the diaphysis. These fractures always involve the articular surface and the metaphysis. In the Groups C1 and C2 the articular surface is split by one fracture line creating only two articular fragments, whereas in the Group C3 the articular surface is split into more than two fragments.

C1 represents simple articular fractures with simple metaphyseal fractures. C2 represents simple articular fractures with a multifragmentary metaphyseal fractures, and C3 represents all multifragmentary articular fractures regardless of the configuration of their metaphyseal fracture.

The C fractures of the **proximal radius/ulna** represent fractures which involve the articular surface of both bones. These are not in the true sense complete articular fractures as one part of the articular surface can retain its continuity with the diaphysis. The Group C1 represents simple articular fractures of both bones, the Group C2 multifragmentary fractures of one articulation and simple of the other, and C3 multifragmentary articular fractures of both bones.

Fig. 20   **The groups C1, C2, C3 of segments 13-, 21-, and 23-**

13- Humerus distal
- C1   Complete articular fracture, articular simple, metaphyseal simple
- C2   Complete articular fracture, articular simple, metaphyseal multifragmentary
- C3   Complete articular fracture, multifragmentary

21- Radius/Ulna proximal
- C1   Articular fracture, of both bones, simple
- C2   Articular fracture, of both bones, the one simple and the other multifragmentary
- C3   Articular fracture, of both bones, multifragmentary

23- Radius/Ulna distal
- C1   Complete articular fracture, of the radius, articular simple, metaphyseal simple
- C2   Complete articular fracture, of the radius, articular simple, metaphyseal multifragmentary
- C3   Complete articular fracture, of the radius, multifragmentary

42

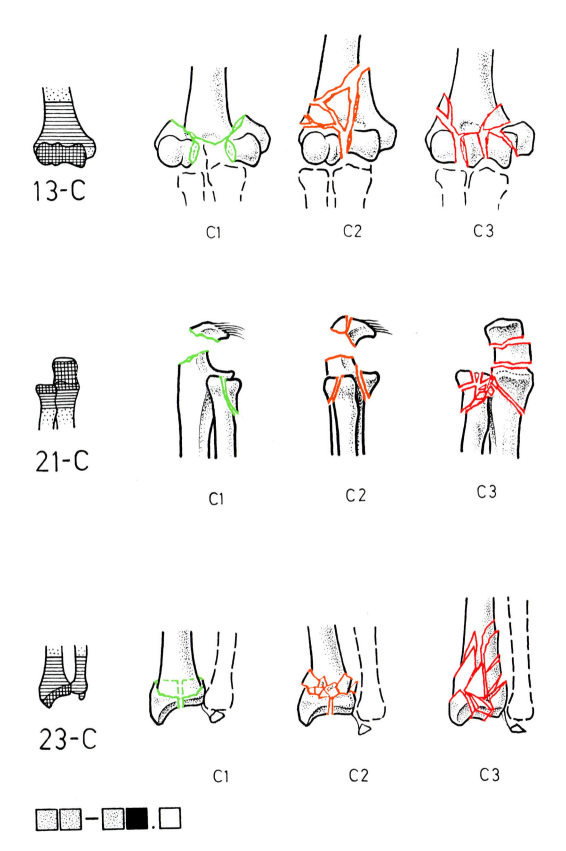

13-C

C1   C2   C3

21-C

C1   C2   C3

23-C

C1   C2   C3

In the **distal femur** the complete articular fractures are classified as follows: C1 represents the articular simple and metaphyseal simple fractures, C2 represents the articular simple and metaphyseal multifragmentary fractures, and C3 the multifragmentary fractures.

In the **proximal tibia/fibula,** the complete articular fractures are classified as follows: C1 represents articular simple and metaphyseal simple fractures, C2 articular simple and metaphyseal multifragmentary fractures, and C3 multifragmentary fractures.

In the **distal tibia/fibula,** complete articular fractures are classified as follows: C1 represents articular simple fractures and metaphyseal simple fractures, C2 represents articular simple fractures and metaphyseal multifragmentary fractures, and C3 multifragmentary fractures.

Fig. 21   **The groups C1, C2, C3 of segments 33-, 41-, and 43-**

33- Femur distal
C1   Complete articular fracture, articular simple, metaphyseal simple
C2   Complete articular fracture, articular simple, metaphyseal multifragmentary
C3   Complete articular fracture, multifragmentary

41- Tibia/Fibula proximal
C1   Complete articular fracture, articular simple, metaphyseal simple
C2   Complete articular fracture, articular simple, metaphyseal multifragmentary
C3   Complete articular fracture, multifragmentary

43- Tibia/Fibula distal
C1   Complete articular fracture, articular simple, metaphyseal simple
C2   Complete articular fracture, articular simple, metaphyseal multifragmentary
C3   Complete articular fracture, multifragmentary

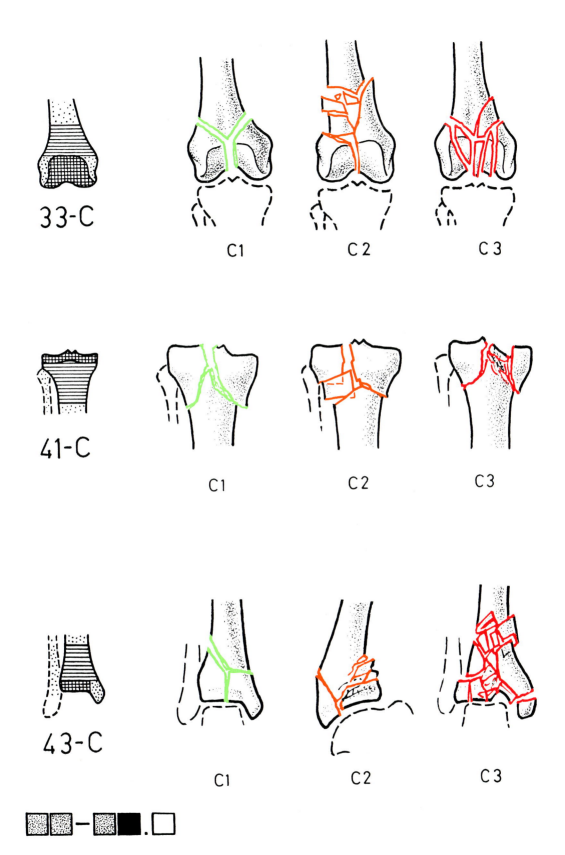

33-C

C1   C2   C3

41-C

C1   C2   C3

43-C

C1   C2   C3

2.4.7   The Nine Groups A1 to C3 of the Proximal Humerus = Segment 11-

In the **proximal humerus**, Type **A** fractures are subdivided as follows: A1 represents isolated tuberosity fractures, A2 impacted metaphyseal fractures, and A3 the metaphyseal fractures without impaction.

The Type **B** fractures are subdivided as follows: B1 represents the tuberosity fractures with impacted metaphyseal fractures, B2 the tuberosity fractures combined with metaphyseal fractures without impaction, and B3 the extra-articular fractures involving a tuberosity and the metaphysis combined with dislocation of the glenohumeral joint.

The Type C fractures, the articular fractures of the proximal humerus, are subdivided as follows: C1 represents the articular fractures through the anatomical neck with slight displacement, C2 the articular fractures through the anatomical neck which are significantly displaced but are impacted and C3 the articular fractures with a glenohumeral dislocation.

Fig. 22   **The nine groups A1 to C3 of the proximal Humerus = segment 11-**

A1	Extra-articular unifocal fracture, tuberosity
A2	Extra-articular unifocal fracture, impacted metaphyseal
A3	Extra-articular unifocal fracture, non-impacted metaphyseal
B1	Extra-articular bifocal fracture, with metaphyseal impaction
B2	Extra-articular bifocal fracture, without metaphyseal impaction
B3	Extra-articular bifocal fracture, with glenohumeral dislocation
C1	Articular fracture, with slight displacement
C2	Articular fracture, impacted with marked displacement
C3	Articular fracture, with glenohumeral dislocation

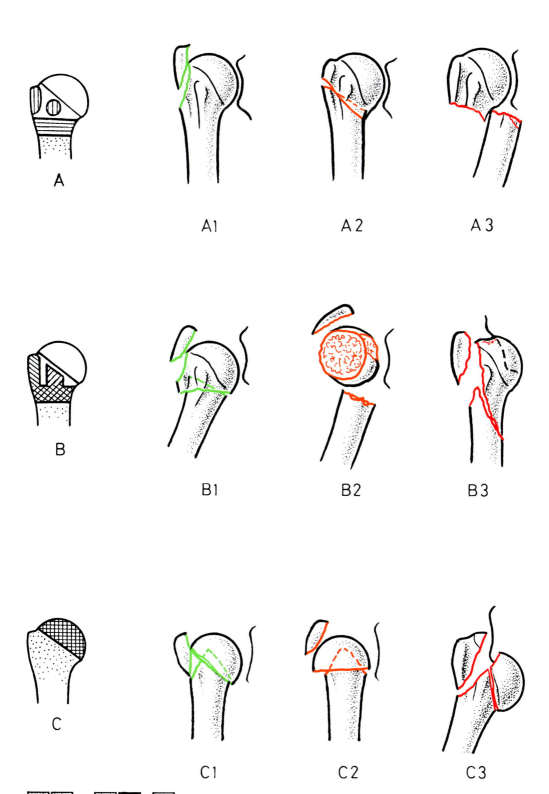

A

A1   A2   A3

B

B1   B2   B3

C

C1   C2   C3

47

2.4.8 The Nine Groups A1 to C3 of the Proximal Femur = Segment 31-

The **proximal femur** is defined by a horizontal line which passes through the inferior border of the lesser trochanter. All fractures with a center at or above this line are thus termed "trochanteric" as long as the fracture line terminates medially above the lesser trochanter.

> **Note:** Subtrochanteric fractures are classified as diaphyseal fractures and appear under the classification for the diaphyseal segment. The dividing line between the subtrochanteric and trochanteric area is a horizontal transverse line at the inferior border of the lesser trochanter.

In the **proximal femur,** the Type **A** fractures are subdivided as follows: A1 represents simple pertrochanteric fractures, A2 multifragmentary pertrochanteric fractures, and A3 true intertrochanteric fractures.

Type **B** fractures are subdivided as follows: B1 represents subcapital fractures with slight displacement, B2 transcervical fractures, and B3 displaced subcapital fractures.

Type **C** represent fractures of the femoral head and are subdivided as follows: C1 represents pure split fractures due to a shearing force, C2 head fractures with depression, and C3 head fractures with neck fracture.

Fig. 23   **The nine groups A1 to C3 of the proximal Femur = segment 31-**

A1	Trochanteric area fracture, pertrochanteric simple
A2	Trochanteric area fracture, pertrochanteric multifragmentary
A3	Trochanteric area fracture, intertrochanteric
B1	Neck fracture, subcapital, with slight displacement
B2	Neck fracture, transcervical
B3	Neck fracture, subcapital, non-impacted, displaced
C1	Head fracture, split
C2	Head fracture, with depression
C3	Head fracture, with neck fracture

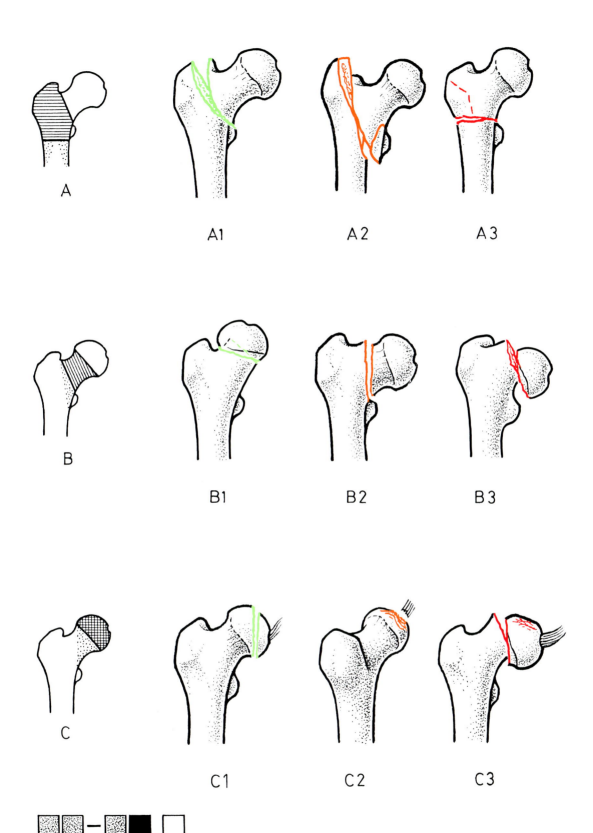

A

A1   A2   A3

B

B1   B2   B3

C

C1   C2   C3

49

2.4.9 The Avulsion Fractures of the Proximal and Distal Segments

As a rule in dealing with the extra-articular fractures (A) it is the degree of instability, the number of fragments and the relative displacement, which determines their classification into the respective subgroups. In partial articular fractures (B) the location of the fracture line and the number of fragments determine their assignment in the subgroup. In complete articular fractures (C) the criterion is a combination of both fractures, extra- and articular, which determines the subdivision.

Avulsion fractures are classified either in the Group A1 (proximal and distal humerus, proximal tibia), or in the Subgroup A1.1 (distal femur, proximal and distal radius/ulna). The rare avulsion fracture of the radial bicipital tuberosity is classified as A2.1.

In the malleolar segment, small avulsion fractures of the lateral and medial malleolus are classified under Type A. Avulsion fractures of the tibio-fibular syndesmotic ligaments are classified under Type B and C. These are the avulsion fractures of the anterior tubercle of Tillaux-Chaput and of the posterior triangle of Volkmann. (See pp. 184-191).

> **Please note:** In the proximal femur the isolated avulsion fractures of the greater and lesser trochanters are classified as Group 31-D1 (as are any fractures which do not fit a group)

Fig. 24   **The avulsion fractures**

11-A1   Humerus proximal, extra-articular unifocal fracture, tuberosity
.1   greater tuberosity not displaced
.2   greater tuberosity displaced
.3   with glenohumeral dislocation
13-A1   Humerus distal, extra-articular fracture, apophyseal avulsion
.1   lateral
.2   medial, non-incarcerated
.3   medial, incarcerated
21-A1   Radius/Ulna proximal, extra-articular fracture of the ulna, radius intact
.1   avulsion of the triceps insertion from the olecranon
21-A2   Radius/Ulna proximal, extra-articular fracture of the radius, ulna intact
.1   avulsion of the bicipital tuberosity of the radius
23-A1   Radius/Ulna distal, extra-articular fracture of the ulna, radius intact
.1   styloid process
33-A1   Femur distal, extra-articular fracture, simple
.1   apophyseal
41-A1   Tibia/Fibula proximal, extra-articular fracture, avulsion
.1   of the fibular head
.2   of the tibial tuberosity
.3   of the intercondylar eminence
44-A   Malleolar segment
A   Lateral infrasyndesmotic lesions: .2 avulsion of the tip of the lateral malleolus
B/C   Lateral transsyndesmotic and suprasyndesmotic fractures of the fibula: avulsions of the tubercle of Chaput and of the Volkmann triangle

11-

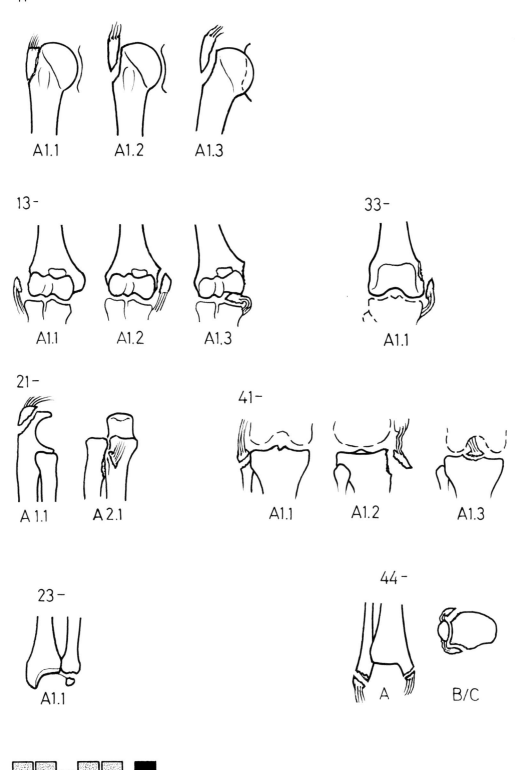

A1.1   A1.2   A1.3

13-

A1.1   A1.2   A1.3

33-

A1.1

21-

A 1.1   A 2.1

41-

A1.1   A1.2   A1.3

23-

A1.1

44-

A   B/C

51

Special Section
Long Bones

1.   Humerus = 1

1.1   Humerus, Proximal Segment = 11-

1.1.1   The Types

Type A reflects the unifocal extra-articular, **Type B** the bifocal extra-articular, and **Type C** the articular fractures.

Unifocal extra-articular fractures involve either one of the tuberosities or the proximal metaphysis of the humerus.

Bifocal extra-articular fractures involve both the metaphysis and one of the tuberosities.

Fig. 25   **Humerus proximal: the bone, the segment, and the types**

        1   Humerus
        11-   Humerus proximal
        11-A Humerus proximal, extra-articular unifocal fracture
        11-B Humerus proximal, extra-articular bifocal fracture
        11-C Humerus proximal, articular fracture

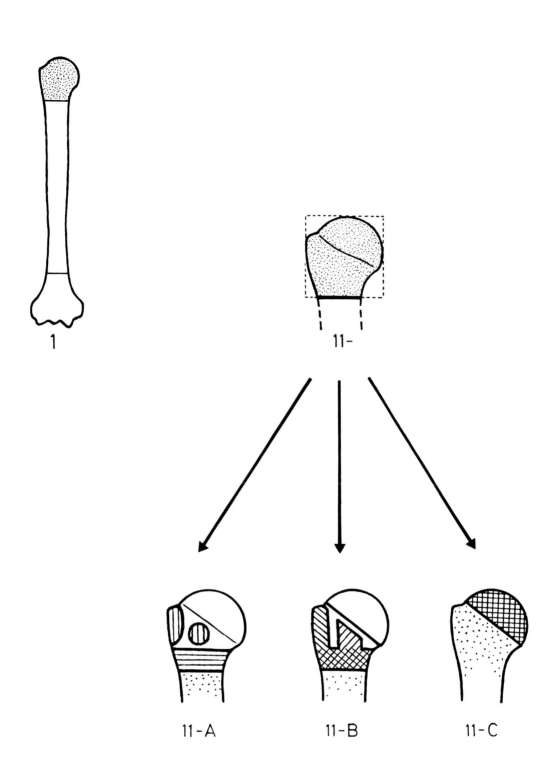

1

11-

11-A   11-B   11-C

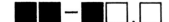

1.1.2 The Groups

The Type A fractures are divided into three groups of increasing severity. **Group A1** are the extra-articular unifocal tuberosity fractures. **Group A2** are the extra-articular unifocal fractures impacted metaphyseal, and **Group A3** are the extra-articular unifocal fractures non-impacted metaphyseal.

The Type B fractures are divided into the three following **groups**: **B1** are the extra-articular bifocal fractures with metaphyseal impaction; **B2** are the extra-articular bifocal fractures without metaphyseal impaction, and **B3** are the extra-articular bifocal fractures with glenohumeral dislocation.

The Type C fractures are articular. The fracture line separates the anatomic head which is completely covered by articular cartilage from the rest of the bone. Occasionally the head itself may be fragmented. The three groups are divided according to the displacement, the impaction of the main fragments and dislocation. Thus the three **groups** are: **C1**, the slightly displaced articular fractures; **C2**, the displaced and impacted articular fractures and **C3**, the dislocated articular fractures.

Please note:
1) The unifocal Type A fractures are considered as extra-articular. It should be noted that a fracture line involving the metaphysis may reach the lowest part of the head. Similarly, a fracture line involving the greater tuberosity, may reach the uppermost part of the head. These features do not impair the articulation. On the other hand, an A1 fracture of the greater tuberosity, if it is displaced or neglected, will result in impairment of shoulder function because of displacement of the rotator cuff insertion and consequent impingement. Despite this risk, such lesions have been classed here because with proper treatment the outcome is usually good.
2) Group B fractures are subject to the same reservations as A1 fractures if they are associated with articular involvement. It must be pointed out, however, that in B1 and B2, the fracture lines involve only the very borders of the articular surface. Articular impairment is more severe in B3 fractures which should be considered as an intermediate pattern between Group B and C fractures.

Fig. 26   **Humerus proximal: the groups**

A1   Extra-articular unifocal fracture, tuberosity
A2   Extra-articular unifocal fracture, impacted metaphyseal
A3   Extra-articular unifocal fracture, non-impacted metaphyseal

B1   Extra-articular bifocal fracture, with metaphyseal impaction
B2   Extra-articluar bifocal fracture, without metaphyseal impaction
B3   Extra-articular bifocal fracture, with glenohumeral dislocation

C1   Articular fracture, with slight displacement
C2   Articular fracture, impacted with marked displacement
C3   Articular fracture, with glenohumeral dislocation

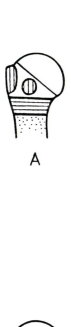

A

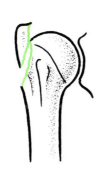

A1

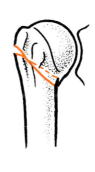

A2

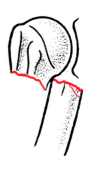

A3

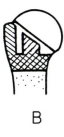

B

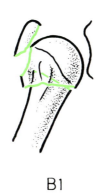

B1

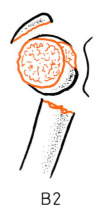

B2

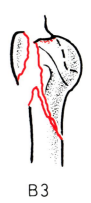

B3

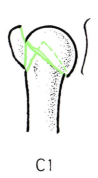

C1

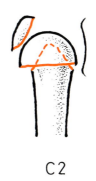

C2

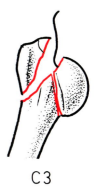

C3

C

57

1.1.3   The Subgroups and Their Qualifications

Fig. 27   **Humerus proximal: the subgroups and their qualifications**

A 1   Extra-articular unifocal fracture, tuberosity
.1   greater tuberosity, not displaced
.2   greater tuberosity, displaced
1) superior   2) posterior
.3   with a glenohumeral dislocation
1) anterior and medial + posterior cephalic notch
2) anterior and medial + greater tuberosity
3) erecta and greater tuberosity   4) posterior and lesser tuberosity

A 2   Extra-articular unifocal fracture, impacted metaphyseal
.1   without frontal malalignment
1) without sagittal malalignment
2) posterior impaction   3) anterior impaction
.2   with varus malalignment
1) pure medial impaction   2) posterior and medial impaction
3) anterior and medial impaction
.3   with valgus malalignment
1) pure lateral impaction   2) posterior and lateral impaction
3) anterior and lateral impaction

A 3   Extra-articular unifocal fracture, non-impacted metaphyseal
.1   simple, with angulation
.2   simple, with translation
1) lateral   2) medial
3) with glenohumeral dislocation
.3   multifragmentary
1) wedge   2) complex
3) with glenohumeral dislocation

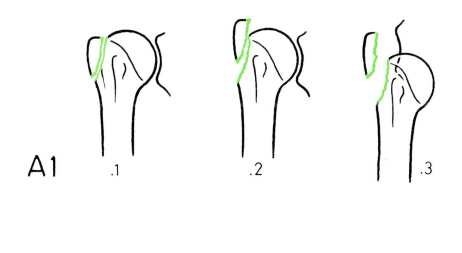

A1

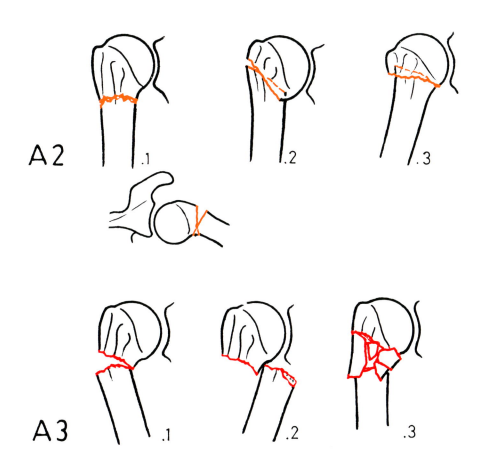

A2

A3

59

The Type B fractures are considered as bifocal because both the metaphysis and the tuberosity are fractured. However, the blood supply to the head is almost never interrupted.

In the **Subgroup B1.1** the fracture of the metaphysis is impacted. The severity of this fracture depends on the degree of impaction of the metaphysis and on the degree of displacement of the greater tuberosity.
The fractures in the **Subgroup B.1.2** have a poorer prognosis. Although less common, they are often associated with a slight varus and downward dislocation of the head.
The **Subgroup B1.3** is included here because of the inherent danger of missing its anterior angulation if only an AP X-ray is taken.

The **B2** Group fractures are unstable because the metaphysis is not impacted. Because of either instability and/or irreducibility, they often require an open reduction and internal fixation.

The **B3** Group fractures are further complicated by dislocation of the head.
The **B3.1** and **B3.2 Subgroups** are very similar. Although in the Subgroup B3.1 there is only a single fracture line, these fractures are classified with the bifocal fractures because the fracture line first crosses the greater tuberosity and then continues through the metaphysis.

Fig. 28   **B1   Extra-articular bifocal fracture, with metaphyseal impaction**
       .1   lateral + greater tuberosity
                1) pure lateral impaction   *2) posterior and lateral impaction*
                3) anterior and lateral impaction
       .2   medial + lesser tuberosity
                1) pure lateral impaction   *2) posterior and lateral impaction*
                3) anterior and lateral impaction
       .3   posterior + greater tuberosity

    B2   Extra-articular bifocal fracture, without metaphyseal impaction
       .1   without rotatory displacement of the epiphyseal fragment
       .2   with rotatory displacement of the epiphyseal fragment
                1) greater tuberosity separated   *2) lesser tuberosity separated*
       .3   multifragmentary metaphyseal + one of the tuberosities
                1) lesser tuberosity   *2) greater tuberosity*

    B3   Extra-articular bifocal fracture, with glenohumeral dislocation
       .1   "vertical" cervical line + greater tuberosity intact + anterior and medial dislocation
       .2   "vertical" cervical line + greater tuberosity fractured + anterior and medial dislocation
       .3   lesser tuberosity fractured + posterior dislocation
                1) without anterior cephalic notch   *2) with anterior cephalic notch*

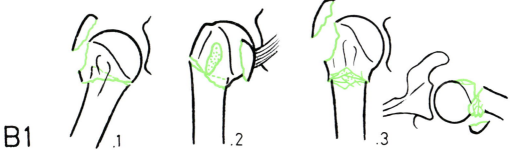

B1

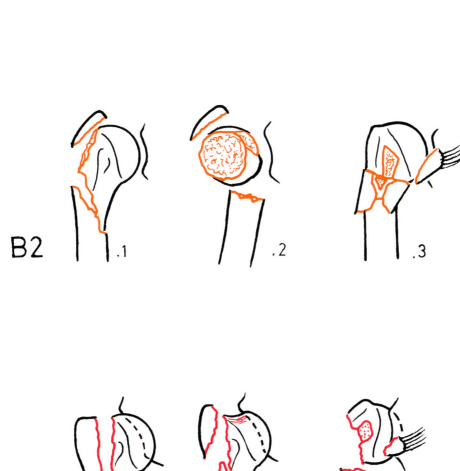

B2

B3

The Type C fractures are articular and involve the anatomic neck of the humerus. Their severity stems from the impairment of the blood supply and the subsequent frequent avascular necrosis of the head.

The Group C1 articular fractures are characterized by their slight displacement. In the **Subgroups C1.1** and **C1.2** both the humeral neck and the tuberosities are involved. In C1.1 the neck fracture is impacted with the head in valgus and in C1.2 with the head in varus. The isolated fractures of the anatomical neck are extremely rare. They have been isolated perhaps somewhat artificially in the **Subgroup C1.3**.

The C2 Group is characterized by marked displacement of the head and by the impaction between the head and the metaphysis. In the **Subgroup C2.1** the head is impacted in valgus and in **C2.2** in varus.

The Group C3 fractures are characterized by the associated dislocation of the head.
The prognosis of the **C3.2** fractures may be better than **C3.1** fractures only in the impacted variety, which is not disimpacted during reduction. It is, however, this feature that makes diagnosis and treatment difficult.
In the **C3.3** fractures not all the head fragments need be necessarily dislocated from the joint.

Fig. 29 **C1** **Articular fracture, with slight displacement**
      .1 cephalotubercular, with valgus malalignment
      .2 cephalotubercular, with varus malalignment
      .3 anatomical neck
          1) non-displaced   *2) displaced*

    C2 **Articular fracture, impacted with marked displacement**
      .1 cephalotubercular, with valgus malalignment
      .2 cephalotubercular, with varus malalignment
      .3 transcephalic (double profile image on X-ray) and tubercular, with varus malalignment

    C3 **Articular fracture, dislocated**
      .1 anatomical neck
          1) anterior   *2) posterior*
      .2 anatomical neck and tuberosities
          1) head impacted   *2) head non-impacted*
      .3 cephalotubercular fragmentation
          1) head intact   *2) head fragmented*

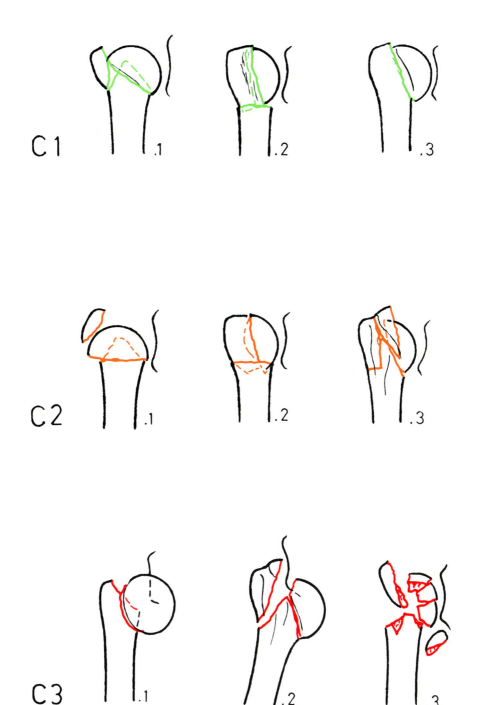

C 1   .1   .2   .3

C 2   .1   .2   .3

C 3   .1   .2   .3

1.2.   Humerus, Diaphyseal Segment = 12-

1.2.1   The Types

Fig. 30   **Humerus diaphysis: the segment, the types**

     12-   Humerus diaphysis
     12-A   Humerus diaphysis, simple fracture
     12-B   Humerus diaphysis, wedge fracture
     12-C   Humerus diaphysis, complex fracture

64

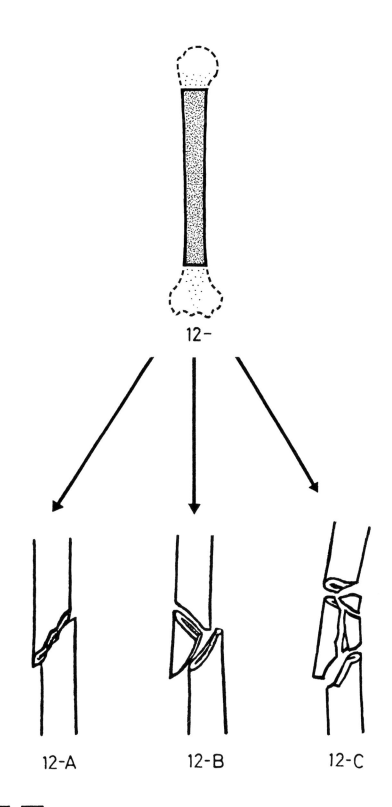

12–

12-A   12-B   12-C

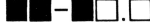

1.2.2 The Groups

Fig. 31 **Humerus diaphysis: the groups**

A1 Simple fracture, spiral
A2 Simple fracture, oblique (≥ 30°)
A3 Simple fracture, transverse (< 30°)

B1 Wedge fracture, spiral wedge
B2 Wedge fracture, bending wedge
B3 Wedge fracture, fragmented wedge

C1 Complex fracture, spiral
C2 Complex fracture, segmental
C3 Complex fracture, irregular

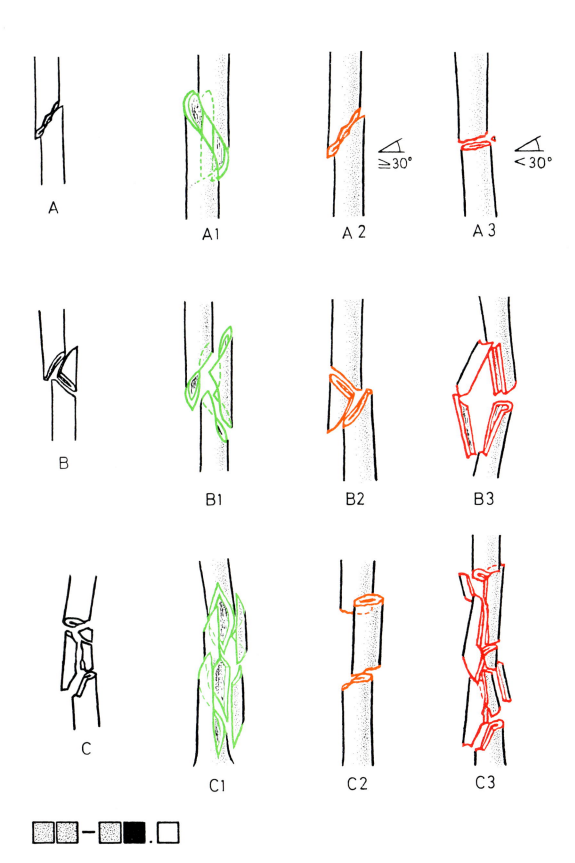

A   A1   A 2   ≧ 30°   A 3   < 30°

B   B1   B2   B3

C   C1   C2   C3

1.2.3   The Subgroups and Their Qualifications

Fig. 32   **Humerus diaphysis: the subgroups and their qualifications**

A 1   Simple fracture, spiral
.1   proximal zone
.2   middle zone
.3   distal zone

A 2   Simple fracture, oblique (≥30°)
.1   proximal zone
.2   middle zone
.3   distal zone

A 3   Simple fracture, transverse (<30°)
.1   proximal zone
.2   middle zone
.3   distal zone

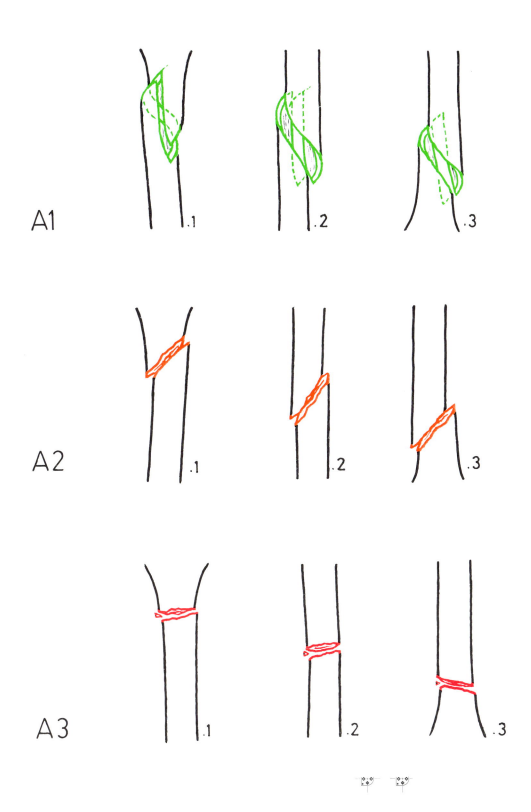

A1

.1　　　　　.2　　　　　.3

A2

.1　　　　　.2　　　　　.3

A3

.1　　　　　.2　　　　　.3

69

Humerus Diaphysis = 12- (Cont.)

Fig. 33   **B1   Wedge fracture, spiral wedge**
.1   proximal zone
.2   middle zone
.3   distal zone

B2   Wedge fracture, bending wedge
.1   proximal zone
.2   middle zone
.3   distal zone

B3   Wedge fracture, fragmented wedge
1) spiral wedge   *2) bending wedge*
.1   proximal zone
.2   middle zone
.3   distal zone

70

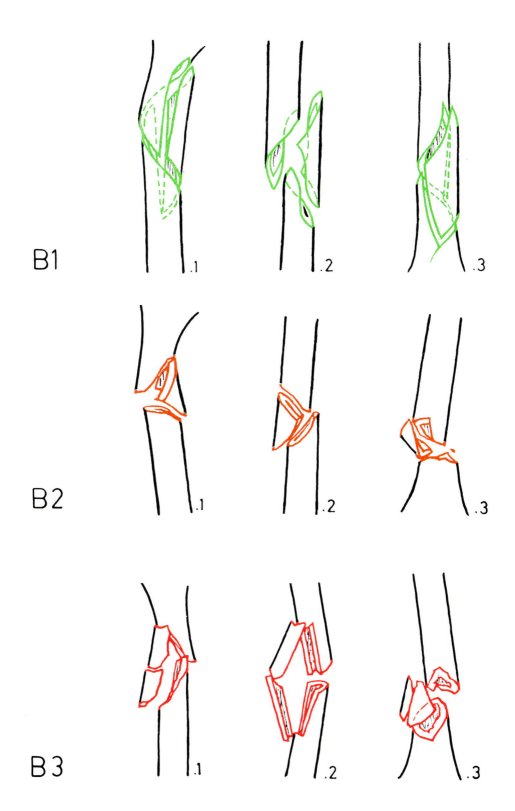

B1   .1   .2   .3

B2   .1   .2   .3

B3   .1   .2   .3

71

Fig. 34   **C 1   Complex fracture, spiral**

1) pure diaphyseal   *2) proximal diaphysio-metaphyseal*
3) distal diaphysio-metaphyseal

   .1   with two intermediate fragments
   .2   with three intermediate fragments
   .3   with more than three intermediate fragments

C 2   Complex fracture, segmental

   .1   with one intermediate segmental fragment

1) pure diaphyseal   *2) proximal diaphysio-metaphyseal*
3) distal diaphysio-metaphyseal   *4) oblique lines*
5) transverse and oblique lines

   .2   with one intermediate segmental and additional wedge fragment(s)

1) pure diaphyseal   *2) proximal diaphysio-metaphyseal*
3) distal diaphysio-metaphyseal   *4) distal wedge*
5) two wedges, proximal and distal

   .3   with two intermediate segmental fragments

1) pure diaphyseal   *2) proximal diaphysio-metaphyseal*
3) distal diaphysio-metaphyseal

C 3   Complex fracture, irregular

   .1   with two or three intermediate fragments

1) two main intermediate fragments
2) three main intermediate fragments

   .2   with limited shattering (< 4 cm)

1) proximal zone   *2) middle zone*
3) distal zone

   .3   with extensive shattering (≥ 4 cm)

1) pure diaphyseal   *2) proximal diaphysio-metaphyseal*
3) distal diaphysio-metaphyseal

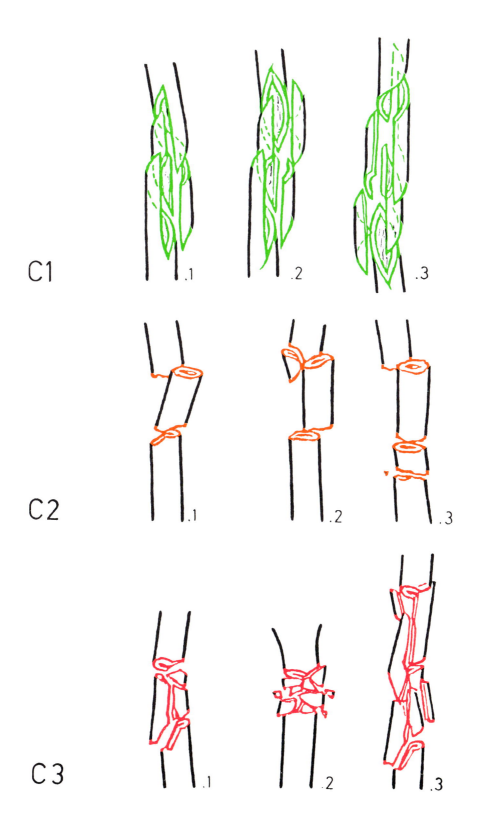

C1   .1   .2   .3

C2   .1   .2   .3

C3   .1   .2   .3

1.3   Humerus, Distal Segment = 13-

The distal segment of the humerus is called the "distal humerus". It is shown within its square (see page 10).

1.3.1   The Types

The fracture types are as follows: – **Type A**: extra-articular fractures; – **Type B**: partial articular fractures; – **Type C**: complete articular fractures.

> **Please note:** Types **B** and **C** comprise fractures with more than two fragments. These can therefore be referred to as **multifragmentary fractures** in distinction to the **simple fractures** Type **A**.

Fig. 35   **Humerus distal: the bone, the segment, and the types**

1	Humerus
13-	Humerus distal
13-A	Humerus distal, extra-articular fracture
13-B	Humerus distal, partial articular fracture
13-C	Humerus distal, complete articular fracture

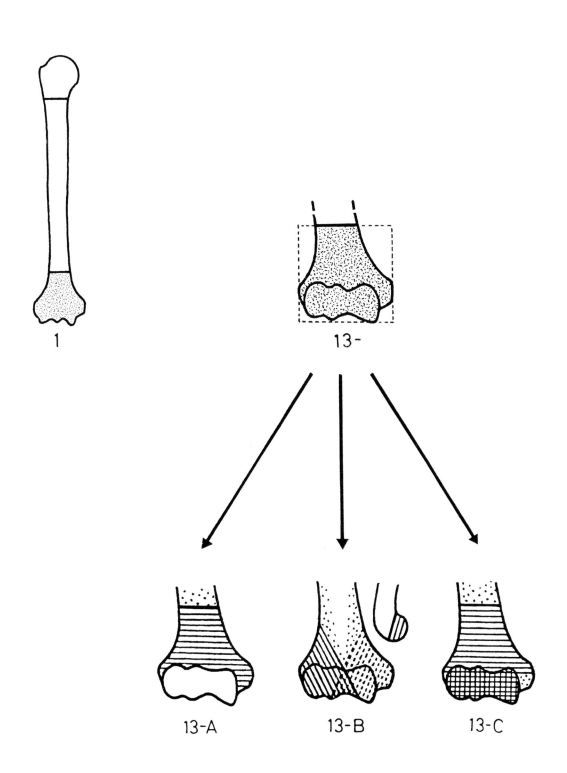

1

13-

13-A   13-B   13-C

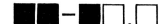

1.3.2 The Groups

The features which we use to separate the Type **A** fractures into their respective groups are first the location of the fracture line (epicondylar or metaphyseal), and secondly whether the fracture of the metaphysis is simple or multifragmentary.

The features which separate the Type B fractures into their respective groups are the direction of the fracture plane (sagittal or frontal) and whether the separated articular fragment is lateral or medial. **Group B1** are the lateral and **Group B2** the medial partial articular fractures. Both fractures are in the sagittal plane and result in a separation of the articular fragment from the rest of the metaphysis. In **Group B3** the fracture line is mainly in the frontal plane and separates a portion of the articular surface from the rest of the joint.

The Type C fractures are classified on the basis of the degree of articular involvement and the degree of metaphyseal fragmentation. Thus in **C1** and **C2**, the articular component of the fracture is simple while in C1 the fracture of the metaphysis is simple and in C2 multifragmentary. All fractures in which the articular component is multi-fragmentary are assigned to **C3** regardless of the state of the metaphyseal component.

Fig. 36   **Humerus distal: the groups**

A1	Extra-articular fracture, apophyseal avulsion
A2	Extra-articular fracture, metaphyseal simple
A3	Extra-articular fracture, metaphyseal multifragmentary
B1	Partial articular fracture, lateral sagittal
B2	Partial articular fracture, medial sagittal
B3	Partial articular fracture, frontal
C1	Complete articular fracture, articular simple, metaphyseal simple
C2	Complete articular fracture, articular simple, metaphyseal multifragmentary
C3	Complete articular fracture, multifragmentary

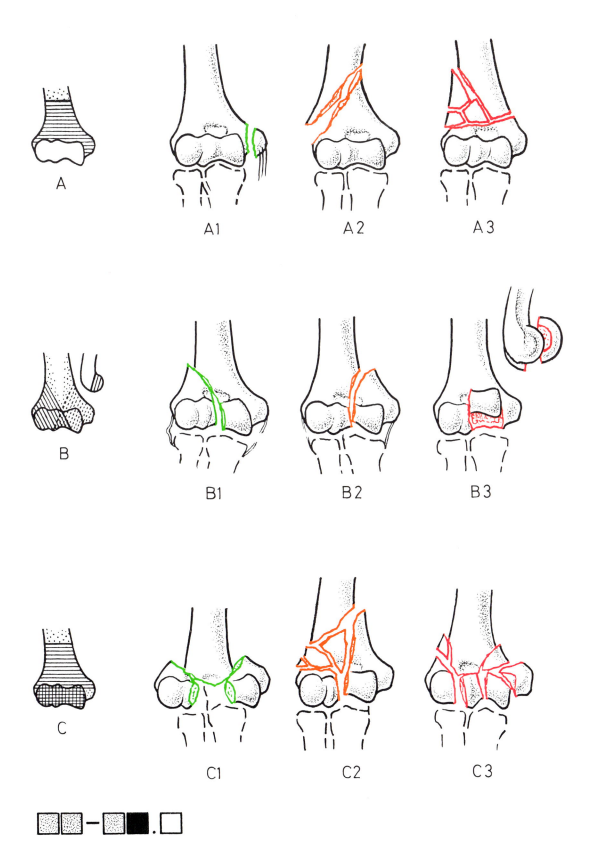

A

A1 A2 A3

B

B1 B2 B3

C

C1 C2 C3

77

1.3.3   The Subgroups and Their Qualifications

The Subgroups of the Group A1, i.e. epicondylar fractures, are classified according to the side involved. The lateral lesions are more accessible surgically. On the medial side there is the added danger of injury to the ulnar nerve. The qualifications (1) and (2) for the **Subgroup A1.2** indicate whether the medial fragment is displaced or not. The qualification (3) indicates that the epicondylar fragment is fragmented.

The Subgroups of the Group A2, i.e. the simple extra-articular metaphyseal fractures, are classified on the basis of the direction of the fracture line. In the **Subgroup A2.1** the sagittal fracture line runs obliquely from proximal and lateral to distal and medial. This results in a lateral displacement of the fragment. Surgical management of these fractures is easier than for **Subgroup A2.2** which has an oblique fracture line which runs downwards and laterally and results in a medial displacement of the fragment. In the **Subgroup A2.3** the fracture line is transverse. The bony lesion may be associated with a vascular or nerve injury due to anterior displacement of the proximal fragment (Kocher I). These fractures are unstable and are almost impossible to manage through an isolated medial or lateral approach.

The Subgroups of the Group A3, i.e. the metaphyseal multifragmentary fractures, are classified according to the number and the extent of the intermediate fragments. Thus, in **Subgroup A3.1** the intermediate wedge is in one piece, in **Subgroup A3.2** the wedge is fragmented, and in **Subgroup A3.3** the metaphyseal fracture is complex. The qualifications (1) and (2) for the Subgroups A3.1 and A3.2 indicate whether the intermediate fragment is lateral or medial.

Fig. 37   **Humerus distal: the subgroups and their qualifications**

A1   **Extra-articular fracture, apophyseal avulsion**
     .1   lateral epicondyle
     .2   medial epicondyle, non-incarcerated
            1) non-displaced   *2) displaced*   *3) fragmented*
     .3   medial epicondyle, incarcerated
A2   **Extra-articular fracture, metaphyseal simple**
     .1   oblique downwards and inwards
     .2   oblique downwards and outwards
     .3   transverse
            1) transmetaphyseal
            2) juxta-epiphyseal with posterior displacement (Kocher I)
            3) juxta-epiphyseal with anterior displacement (Kocher II)
A3   **Extra-articular fracture, metaphyseal multifragmentary**
     .1   with an intact wedge
            1) lateral   *2) medial*
     .2   with a fragmented wedge
            1) lateral   *2) medial*
     .3   complex

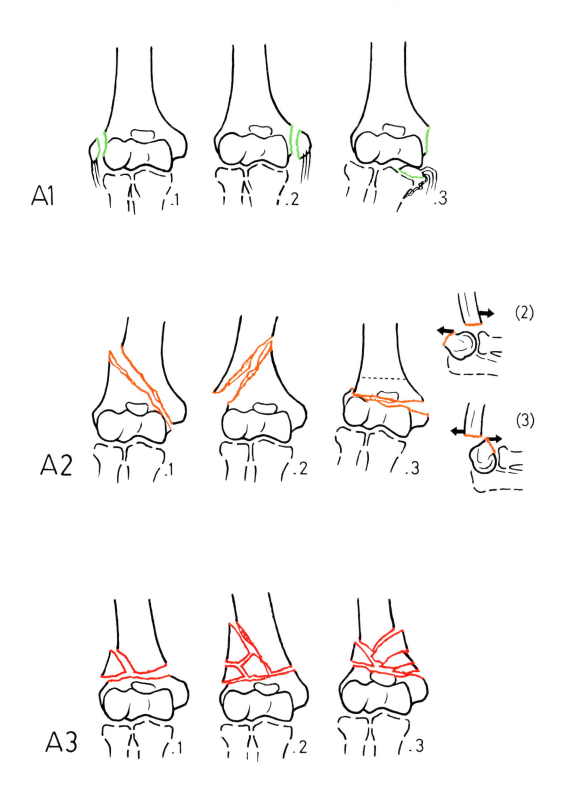

A1 .1 .2 .3

A2 .1 .2 .3 (2) (3)

A3 .1 .2 .3

79

The partial **B1** (lateral) and partial **B2** (medial) articular fractures are classified into **subgroups** according to the size and the number of the articular fragments. Thus in the Subgroups .1 and .2 the detached fragment is intact whereas in Subgroup .3 it is fragmented.

The partial articular **B3** fractures in which the fracture line runs in the frontal plane are classified into subgroups according to the side from which the articular fragment has broken off. Thus in the Subgroup .1 the fragment is from the capitellum, in the Subgroup .2 from the trochlea and in the Subgroup .3 both the capitellum and the trochlea are detached and split apart.

Fig. 38   **B1**   **Partial articular fracture, lateral sagittal**
          .1   capitellum
                1) through the capitellum (Milch I)
                2) between the capitellum and the trochlea
          .2   transtrochlear simple
                1) collateral ligament intact
                2) collateral ligament ruptured
                3) metaphyseal simple (= "classic lateral condyle", Milch II)
                4) metaphyseal wedge
                5) metaphysio-diaphyseal
          .3   transtrochlear multifragmentary
                1) epiphysio-metaphyseal   *2) epiphysio-metaphysio-diaphyseal*

       B2   **Partial articular fracture, medial sagittal**
          .1   transtrochlear simple, through the medial side (Milch I)
          .2   transtrochlear simple, through the groove
                1) collateral ligament intact
                2) collateral ligament ruptured
                3) metaphyseal simple (= "classic medial condyle", Milch II)
                4) metaphyseal wedge   *5) metaphysio-diaphyseal*
          .3   transtrochlear multifragmentary
                1) epiphysio-metaphyseal   *2) epiphysio-metaphysio-diaphyseal*

       B3   **Partial articular fracture, frontal**
          .1   capitellum
                1) incomplete (Kocher-Lorenz)   *2) complete (Hahn-Steinthal 1)*
                3) with a trochlear component (Hahn-Steinthal 2)
                4) fragmented
          .2   trochlea
                1) simple   *2) fragmented*
          .3   capitellum and trochlea

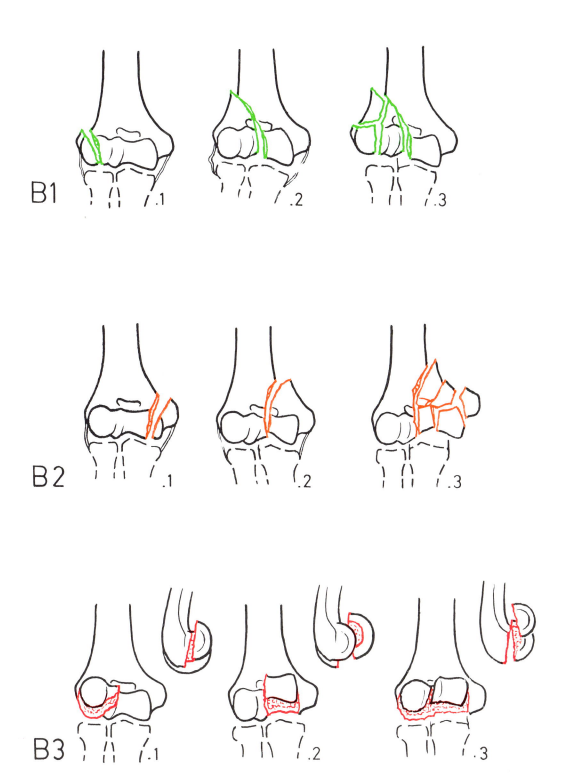

B1   .1   .2   .3

B2   .1   .2   .3

B3   .1   .2   .3

The Type C fractures, i.e. complete articular fractures, are classified according to the pattern of their articular and metaphyseal components.

C1 includes the simple articular and simple metaphyseal fractures. The **subgroups** are distinguished from each other either by the displacement of the fragments or the level of the metaphyseal component. The difference between Subgroups .1 and .2 is the degree of the displacement of the articular fragments. The Subgroup .3 is characterized by the level of the metaphyseal fracture which is very low and passes along the upper edge of the articular surface.

C2 includes the simple articular and multifragmentary metaphyseal fractures. The **subgroups** are distinguished from each other by the number of the metaphyseal fragments and the extent of the fracture.and extent of metaphyseal fragments. Thus in the Subgroup .1 the metaphyseal fragment is an intact wedge, in the Subgroup .2 the metaphyseal wedge is fragmented and in the Subgroup .3 the metaphyseal fracture is complex .

C3 includes the multifragmentary articular fractures regardless of the pattern of the metaphyseal component. The **subgroups** are distinguished from each other on the basis of the extent of metaphyseal fragmentation.

Fig. 39   **C1   Complete articular fracture, articular simple, metaphyseal simple**
　　　　　.1   with slight displacement
　　　　　　　　1) Y-shaped   2) T-shaped metaphyseal   3) V-shaped
　　　　　.2   with marked displacement
　　　　　　　　1) Y-shaped   2) T-shaped metaphyseal   3) V-shaped
　　　　　.3   T-shaped epiphyseal

　　　　C2   Complete articular fracture, articular simple, metaphyseal multifragmentary
　　　　　.1   with an intact wedge
　　　　　　　　1) metaphyseal lateral　　　　　*2) metaphyseal medial*
　　　　　　　　3) metaphysio-diaphyseal lateral　*4) metaphysio-diaphyseal medial*
　　　　　.2   with a fragmented wedge
　　　　　　　　1) metaphyseal lateral　　　　　*2) metaphyseal medial*
　　　　　　　　3) metaphysio-diaphyseal lateral　*4) metaphysio-diaphyseal medial*
　　　　　.3   complex

　　　　C3   Complete articular fracture, multifragmentary
　　　　　.1   metaphyseal simple
　　　　　.2   metaphyseal wedge
　　　　　　　　1) intact　　　　　　　　*2) fragmented*
　　　　　.3   metaphyseal complex
　　　　　　　　1) localized　　　　　　　*2) extending into the diaphysis*

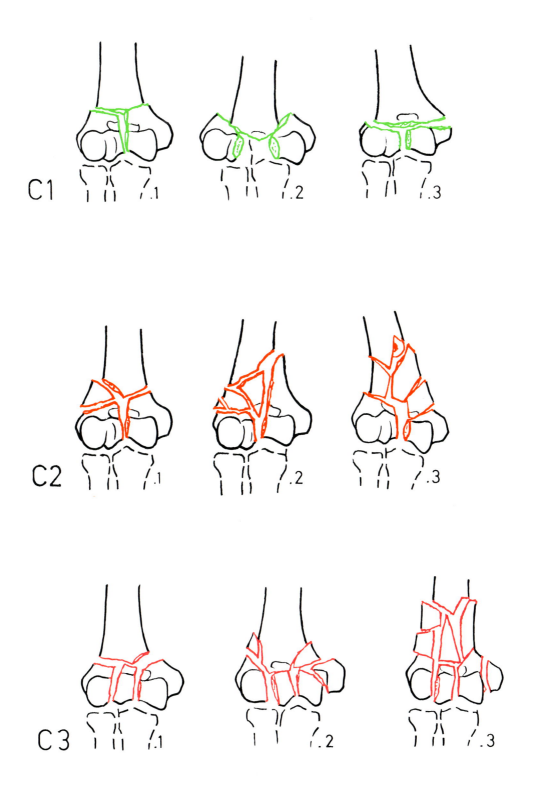

C1   .1   .2   .3

C2   .1   .2   .3

C3   .1   .2   .3

1.3.4   Comments: A comparison of the AO classification of fractures of the distal segment of the humerus with the published classifications.

In 1853, *Hahn* reported a complete fracture of the capitellum with an extension into the trochlea: *Hahn-Steinthal-Fracture* (B3.1(3)). In 1896, *Kocher* described a low transverse metaphyseal fracture associated with either an "anterior or posterior displacement of the shaft" (A2.3). In 1964, *Milch* distinguished two forms of partial articular fractures associated with ligament rupture, i.e. the "classic external condyle" (B1.2), and medially through the groove, the "classic internal condyle" (B2.2). In 1964, *Judet* classified fractures of the distal end of the humerus into 5 groups: 1). complete articular multifragmentary (C3); 2) lateral epicondylar fracture (A1.1); 3) articular simple and metaphyseal simple (C1); 4) medial and lateral partial articular fracture (B2.2 and B1.2); and the simple transverse metaphyseal fracture (A2). In 1969, *Riseborough* and *Radin* described 4 types of fractures of the distal end of the humerus which in their view determined the choice of treatment. The 4 types are the complete articular simple and metaphyseal simple undisplaced and with slight displacement C1.1, with marked displacement C1.2, and the complete articular multifragmentary fracture C3.1

The most complete classification of distal humerus fractures was presented in 1980 at the SOFCOT by *Lecestre et al.* This classification included 10 groups based on 10 basic fracture types which correspond to our coding as follows:

- simple extra-articular shaft fracture with an oblique line running obliquely downward and outward = A2.2;
- simple, transtrochlear, lateral partial articular fracture = B1.2;
- simple, transtrochlear, medial partial articular fracture through the trochlear groove = B2.2;
- simple metaphyseal and simple condylar, total articular fracture with slight displacement = C1.1;
- multifragmentary, total articular fracture = C3.2;
- simple condylar and multifragmentary metaphyseal total articular fracture, with a fragmented metaphyseal wedge = C2.2;
- simple metaphyseal and simple condylar, T-shaped total articular fracture = C1.3;
- simple transverse extra-articular fracture with posterior displacement = A2.3 (2);
- partial articular fracture of the capitellum in the frontal plane with trochlear involvement = B3.1(3);
- partial articular frontal fracture of the capitellum without fragmentation = B3.1(2).

As shown in this review of the literature, the classification systems proposed till now **did not take into account the severity of the fracture.** The system of *Riseborough* and *Radin* is an exception but it includes only subgroups C1.1, C1.2, and C3.1.

Fig. 40   A comparison of the AO classification of fractures of the distal segment of the humerus with the published classifications

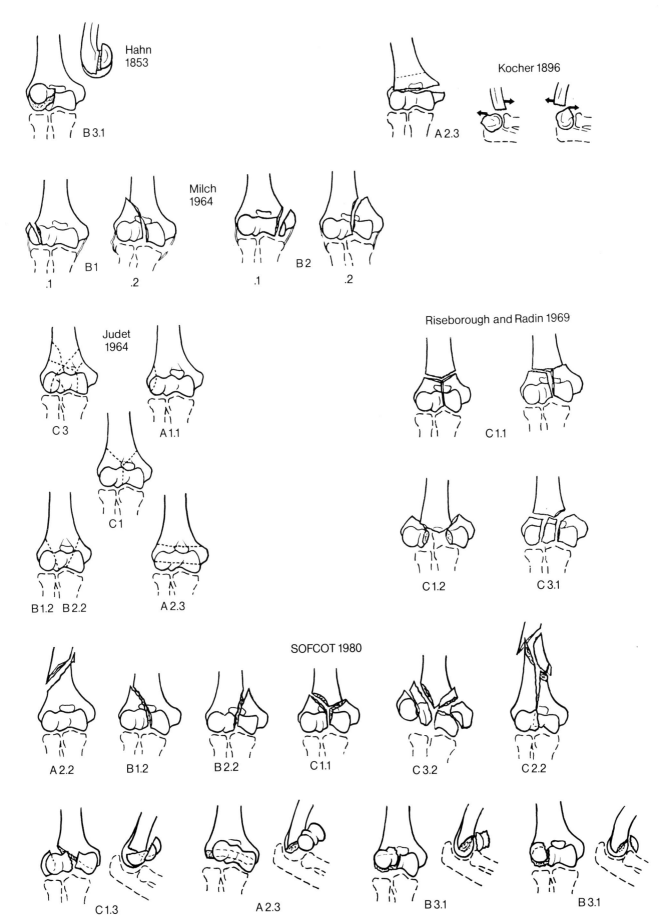

Hahn
1853

B 3.1

Kocher 1896

A 2.3

Milch
1964

B 1

.1   .2

B 2

.1   .2

Judet
1964

C 3   A 1.1

C 1

B 1.2   B 2.2   A 2.3

Riseborough and Radin 1969

C 1.1

C 1.2   C 3.1

SOFCOT 1980

A 2.2   B 1.2   B 2.2   C 1.1   C 3.2   C 2.2

C 1.3   A 2.3   B 3.1   B 3.1

2. Radius/Ulna = 2

2.1 Radius/Ulna, Proximal Segment = 21-

2.1.1 The Types

Fig. 41   **Radius/Ulna proximal: the bones, the segment, and the types**

  2   Radius/Ulna
  21-   Radius/Ulna proximal
  21-A Radius/Ulna proximal , extra-articular fracture
  21-B Radius/Ulna proximal, articular fractures involving the articular surface of only one of
        the two bones
  21-C Radius/Ulna proximal, articular fractures involving the articular surface of both bones

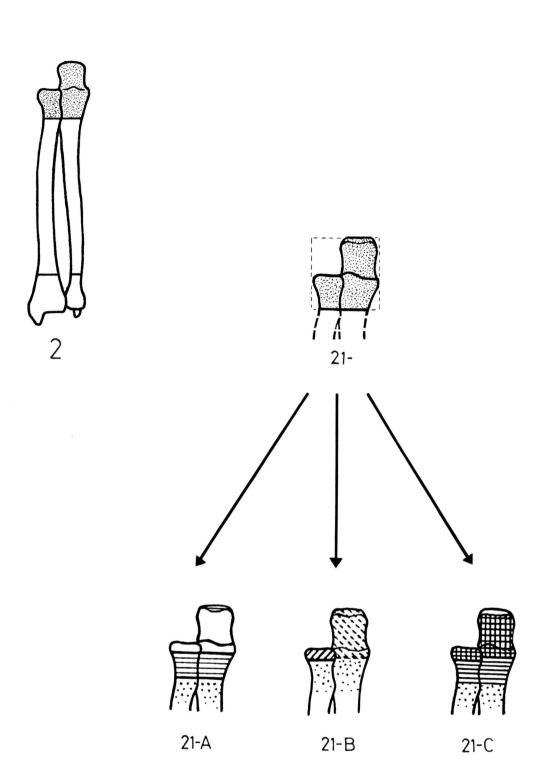

2

21-

21-A   21-B   21-C

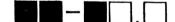

2.1.2 The Groups

As explained previously (see pages 34, 38, and 42), the presence of two bones in the forearm led to a modification of the classification system. In fractures of the proximal segment the two bones are considered as a single articulation with the radius being the lateral and the ulna the medial compartment.

The Type A fractures are extra-articular. The classification depends on the bone involved. Thus fractures of the ulna alone are **A1**, of the radius alone **A2** and of both bones **A3**.

The Type B fractures are partial articular fractures involving the articular surface of only one of the two bones. Thus the **Group B1** are the articular fractures of the ulna with the radius intact, the **Group B2** are the articular fractures of the radius with the ulna intact, and the **Group B3** fractures are the articular fractures of one of the two bones with an extra-articular fracture of the other one.

The Type C fractures are complete articular fractures, which means in this location that the articular surface of both bones is involved. The **C1 Group** includes simple articular fractures of both bones, **C2** simple articular fracture of one and multifragmentary of the other, and **C3** the articular multifragmentary fractures of both bones.

Fig. 42 **Radius/Ulna proximal: the groups**

A1 Extra-articular fracture, of the ulna, radius intact
A2 Extra-articular fracture, of the radius, ulna intact
A3 Extra-articular fracture, of both bones

B1 Articular fracture, of the ulna, radius intact
B2 Articular fracture, of the radius, ulna intact
B3 Articular fracture, of the one bone, extra-articular fracture of the other

C1 Articular fracture, of both bones, simple
C2 Articular fracture, of both bones, the one simple and the other multifragmentary
C3 Articular fracture, of both bones, multifragmentary

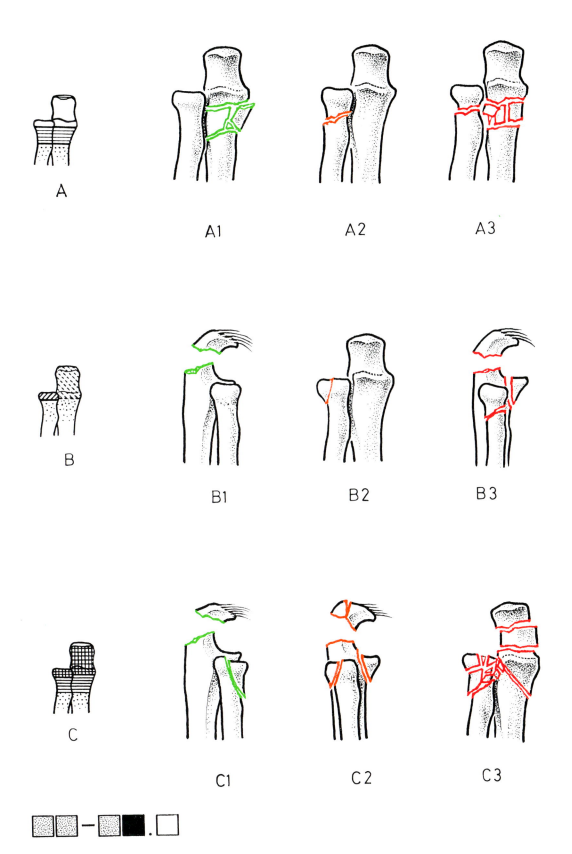

A

A1   A2   A3

B

B1   B2   B3

C

C1   C2   C3

89

2.1.3   The Subgroups and Their Qualifications

Fig. 43   **Radius/Ulna proximal: the subgroups and their qualifications**

A1   Extra-articular fracture, of the ulna, radius intact
.1   avulsion of the triceps insertion from the olecranon
.2   metaphyseal simple
.3   metaphyseal multifragmentary

A2   Extra-articular fracture, of the radius, ulna intact
.1   avulsion of the bicipital tuberosity of the radius
.2   neck simple
.3   neck multifragmentary

A3   Extra-articular fracture, of both bones
.1   simple of both bones
.2   multifragmentary of the one bone and simple of the other
     1) ulna multifragmentary   2) radius multifragmentary
.3   multifragmentary of both bones

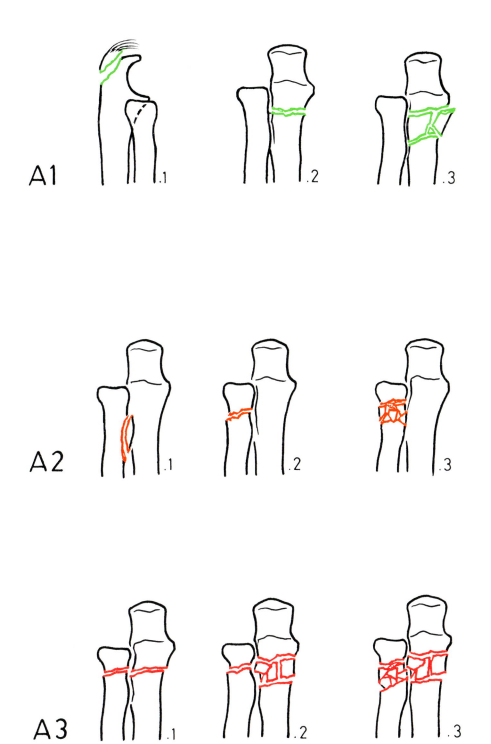

A1   .1   .2   .3

A2   .1   .2   .3

A3   .1   .2   .3

Fig. 44 **B1** **Articular fracture, of the ulna, radius intact**
  .1 unifocal
    1) olecranon one line *2) olecranon two lines*
    3) olecranon multifragmentary *4) coronoid process alone*
  .2 bifocal simple
  .3 bifocal multifragmentary
    1) multifragmentary of the olecranon
    2) multifragmentary of the coronoid process
    3) multifragmentary of both, the olecranon and the coronoid process

  B2 **Articular fracture, of the radius, ulna intact**
  .1 simple
    1) non-displaced *2) displaced*
  .2 multifragmentary without depression
  .3 multifragmentary with depression

  B3 **Articular fracture, of the one bone with extra-articular fracture of the other**
  .1 ulna, articular simple
    1) radius extra-articular simple *2) radius extra-articular multifragmentary*
  .2 radius, articular simple
    1) ulna extra-articular simple *2) ulna extra-articular multifragmentary*
  .3 articular multifragmentary
    1) ulna, radius extra-articular simple
    2) ulna, radius extra-articular multifragmentary
    3) radius, ulna extra-articular simple
    4) radius, ulna extra-articular multifragmentary

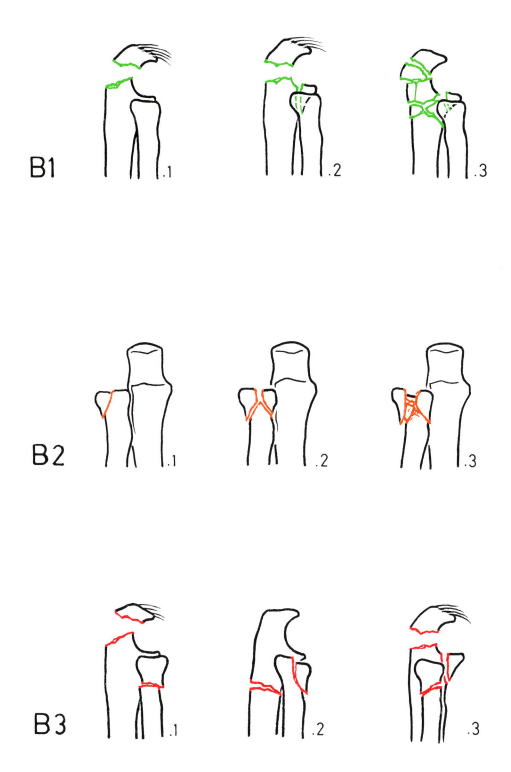

B1   .1   .2   .3

B2   .1   .2   .3

B3   .1   .2   .3

Fig. 45 **C1 Articular fracture, of both bones, simple**
      .1   olecranon and head of radius
      .2   coronoid process and head of radius

      C2 Articular fracture, of both bones, the one simple and the other multifragmentary
      .1   olecranon multifragmentary, radial head simple
      .2   olecranon simple, radial head multifragmentary
      .3   coronoid process simple, radial head multifragmentary

      C3 Articular fracture, of both bones, multifragmentary
      .1   three fragments of each bone
      .2   ulna, more than three fragments
              1) radius, three fragments   *2) radius, more than three fragments*
      .3   radius, more than three fragments
              1) ulna, three fragments   *2) ulna, epiphysio-diaphyseal*

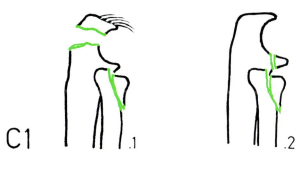

C1

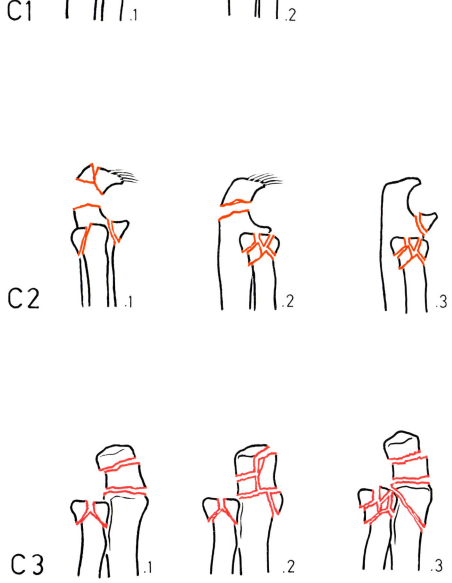

C2

C3

2.2   Radius/Ulna, Diaphyseal Segment = 22-

2.2.1   The Types

The classification of fracture types is based on the same principle for the diaphysis of the radius and the ulna as for other long bones.

Fig. 46   **Radius/Ulna diaphysis: the segment, the types**

22-   Radius/Ulna diaphysis
22-A   Radius/Ulna diaphysis, simple fracture
22-B   Radius/Ulna diaphysis, wedge fracture
22-C   Radius/Ulna diaphysis, complex fracture

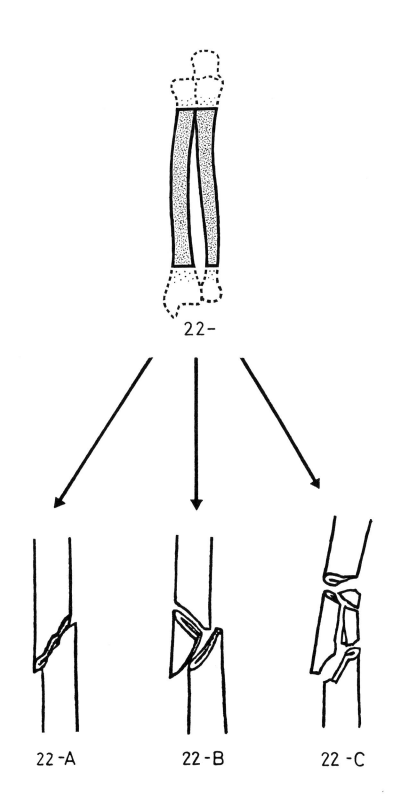

22-

22-A   22-B   22-C

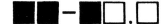

2.2.2   The Groups

The groups are differentiated from each other by the bone involved (radius and/or ulna), rather than by the morphology of the fracture. Surgical management of ulnar lesions is generally easier because of the architecture of the ulna and the superficial location of this bone. This is why in each type, fractures of the ulna are considered as the less severe and ranked in the first position (A1, B1, and C1) while those of the radius are placed in the second position (A2, B2, and C2), and those of both bones in the third (A3, B3, and C3).

Fig. 47   **Radius/Ulna diaphysis: the groups**

A1   Simple fracture, of the ulna, radius intact
A2   Simple fracture, of the radius, ulna intact
A3   Simple fracture, of both bones

B1   Wedge fracture, of the ulna, radius intact
B2   Wedge fracture, of the radius, ulna intact
B3   Wedge fracture, of the one bone, simple or wedge fracture of the other

C1   Complex fracture, of the ulna
C2   Complex fracture, of the radius
C3   Complex fracture, of both bones

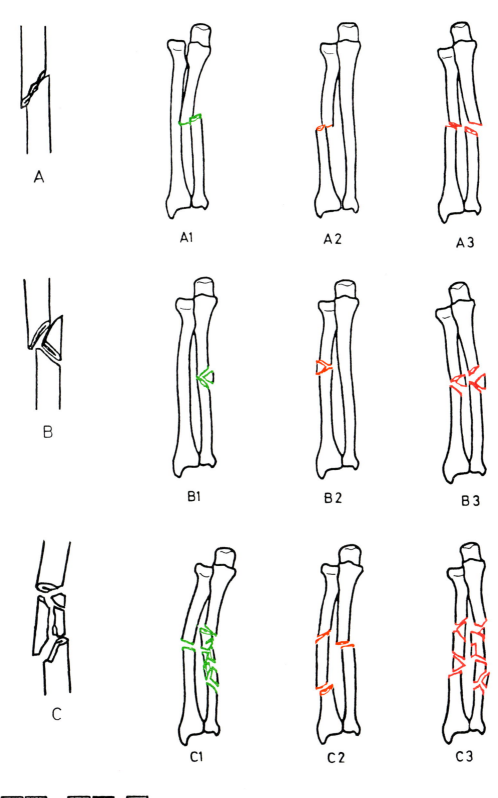

A

A1   A2   A3

B

B1   B2   B3

C

C1   C2   C3

99

2.2.3   The Subgroups and Their Qualifications

The **subgroups of** the **Groups A1** and **A2** are classified on the basis of the direction of the fracture line as well as on the possible concomitant involvement of the radio-ulnar articulations. The Subgroup .1 includes oblique (or spiral) fractures, the Subgroup .2 includes transverse fractures, and the Subgroup .3 includes fractures of one of the bones associated with a dislocation of the proximal or distal radio-ulnar joints (*Monteggia* and *Galeazzi*).

The **subgroups of A3** are determined on the basis of the level of the fracture of the radius.

Fig. 48   **Radius/Ulna diaphysis: the subgroups and their qualifications**

A 1   Simple fracture, of the ulna, radius intact
.1   oblique
.2   transverse
.3   with dislocation of the radial head (Monteggia)

A 2   Simple fracture, of the radius, ulna intact
.1   oblique
.2   transverse
.3   with dislocation of the distal radio-ulnar joint (Galeazzi)

A 3   Simple fracture, of both bones
1) without dislocation
2) with dislocation of the radial head (Monteggia)
3) with dislocation of the distal radio-ulnar joint (Galeazzi)
.1   radius, proximal zone
.2   radius, middle zone
.3   radius, distal zone

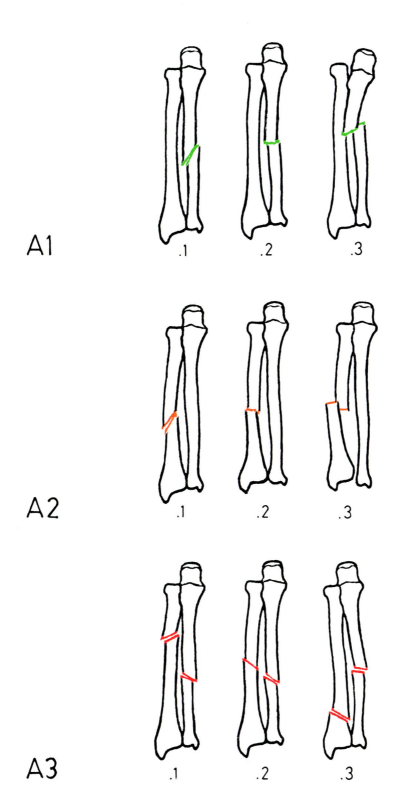

A1
    .1   .2   .3

A2
    .1   .2   .3

A3
    .1   .2   .3

The **subgroups of B1** and **B2** are distinguished from each other on the basis of the condition of the wedge fragment, that is whether it is intact or fragmented, and whether the proximal or distal radio-ulnar joint is dislocated or not. Thus in the Subgroup .1 the wedge is intact, in .2 the wedge is fragmented, and in .3 the wedge fracture of the radius or the ulna is associated with a dislocation of the proximal or distal radio-ulnar joint.

The **B3 subgroups** are classified on the basis of which bone contains the wedge fragment. Thus in the Subgroup .1 the wedge fracture involves the ulna, in .2 the radius, and in .3 both the radius and the ulna.

Fig. 49   **B1   Wedge fracture, of the ulna, radius intact**
.1   intact wedge
.2   fragmented wedge
.3   with dislocation of the radial head (Monteggia)

B2   Wedge fracture, of the radius, ulna intact
.1   intact wedge
.2   fragmented wedge
.3   with dislocation of the distal radio-ulnar joint (Galeazzi)

B3   Wedge fracture, of the one bone, simple or wedge fracture of the other
1) without dislocation
2) with dislocation of the radial head (Monteggia)
3) with dislocation of the distal radio-ulnar joint (Galeazzi)
.1   ulnar wedge and simple fracture of the radius
.2   radial wedge and simple fracture of the ulna
.3   radial and ulnar wedges

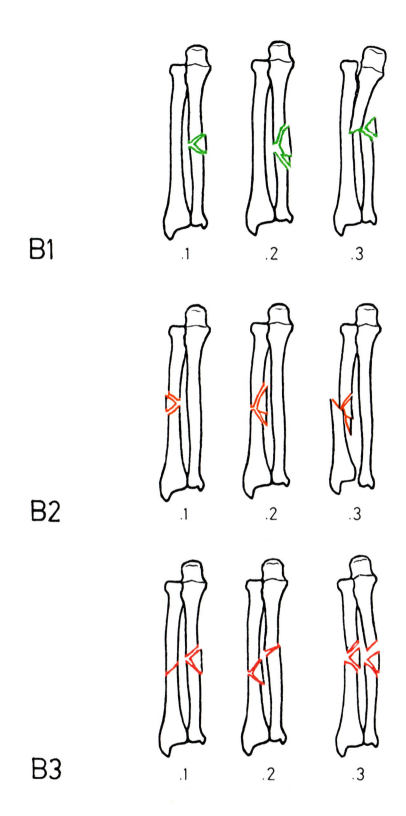

B1

     .1   .2   .3

B2

     .1   .2   .3

B3

     .1   .2   .3

Fig. 50   **C 1**   **Complex fracture, of the ulna**
            .1   bifocal, radius intact
                  1) without dislocation
                  2) with dislocation of the radial head (Monteggia)
            .2   bifocal, radius fractured
                  1) simple   *2) wedge*
            .3   irregular
                  1) radius intact   *2) radius simple*
                  3) radial wedge

        C 2   **Complex fracture, of the radius**
            .1   bifocal, ulna intact
                  1) without dislocation
                  2) with dislocation of the distal radio-ulnar joint (Galeazzi)
            .2   bifocal, ulna fractured
                  1) simple   *2) wedge*
            .3   irregular
                  1) ulna intact   2) ulna simple   3) ulnar wedge

        C 3   **Complex fracture, of both bones**
            .1   bifocal
            .2   bifocal of the one, irregular of the other
                  1) bifocal of radius, irregular of ulna
                  2) bifocal of ulna, irregular of radius
            .3   irregular

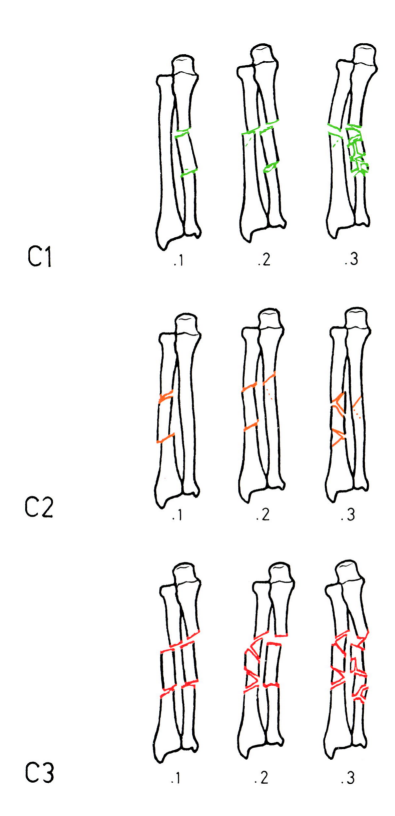

C1   .1   .2   .3

C2   .1   .2   .3

C3   .1   .2   .3

2.3   Radius/Ulna, Distal Segment = 23-

2.3.1   The Types

The fracture types consist of extra-articular fractures (**Type A**), partial articular fractures of the radius (**Type B**), and complete articular fractures of the radius (**Type C**). Isolated extra-articular fractures of the ulna are classified with similar fractures of the radius as Type A.

Fig. 51   **Radius/Ulna distal: the bones, the segment, and the types**

2   Radius/Ulna
23-   Radius/Ulna distal
23-A   Radius/Ulna distal, extra-articular fracture
23-B   Radius/Ulna distal, partial articular fracture of the radius
23-C   Radius/Ulna distal, complete articular fracture of the radius

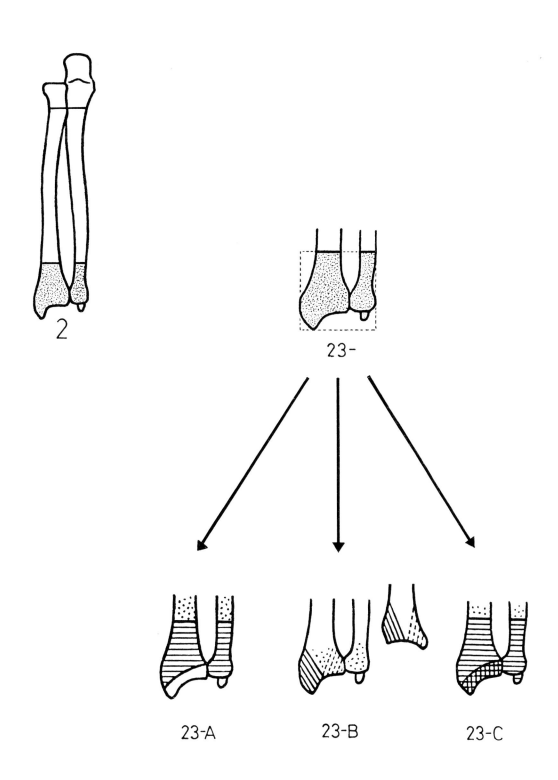

2

23-

23-A   23-B   23-C

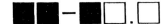

2.3.2 The Groups

The **A1 Group** represents the isolated fractures of the distal metaphysis of the ulna. **A2** and **A3** represent fractures of the distal metaphysis of the radius and are distinguished from each other on the basis of whether the fractures are simple or multifragmentary. Thus in A2 the fracture is simple and in A3 it is multifragmentary.

The groups of Type B, i.e. partial articular fractures, are classified according to the direction of the fracture plane. In the **Group B1**, the fracture plane is sagittal. In the **Group B2**, it is frontal and oblique and runs upwards and backwards and results in the detachment of a dorsal wedge. In the **Group B3**, it is frontal and oblique and runs upwards and forwards and results in the detachment of a volar wedge. The resulting displacement of the carpus is posterior (or dorsal) in B2 and anterior (or volar) in B3.

The groups of Type C, i.e. complete articular fractures, are classified according to whether the articular and metaphyseal components are simple or multifragmentary. In **Group C1**, both the articular and metaphyseal components are simple. In **Group C2**, the articular component is simple and the metaphyseal multifragmentary, and in **Group C3**, the articular component is multifragmentary regardless of the state of the metaphysis.

Fig. 52 **Radius/Ulna distal: the groups**

A1   Extra-articular fracture, of the ulna , radius intact
A2   Extra-articular fracture, of the radius, simple and impacted
A3   Extra-articular fracture, of the radius, multifragmentary

B1   Partial articular fracture, of the radius, sagittal
B2   Partial articular fracture, of the radius, dorsal rim (Barton)
B3   Partial articular fracture, of the radius , volar rim (reverse Barton, Goyrand- Smith II)

C1   Complete articular fracture, of the radius, articular simple, metaphyseal simple
C2   Complete articular fracture, of the radius, articular simple, metaphyseal multifragmentary
C3   Complete articular fracture, of the radius, multifragmentary

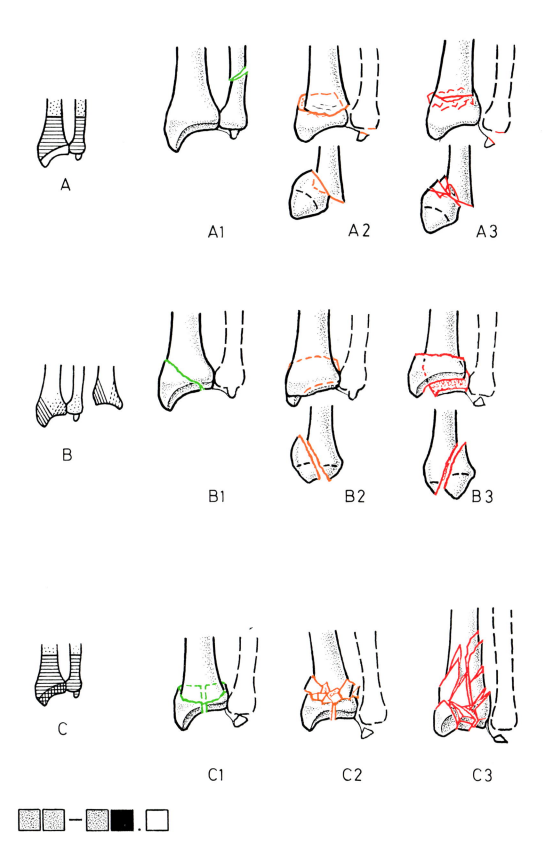

A

A1

A2

A3

B

B1

B2

B3

C

C1

C2

C3

109

2.3.3 The Subgroups and Their Qualifications

The **subgroups of A1** are differentiated on the basis of the fracture patterns of the distal ulna.

The **subgroups of A2** are differentiated on the basis of the direction of the fracture line and of the displacement of the distal fragment. In the Subgroup .1 the fracture line is more or less transverse and the displacement is minimal or axial (compressive axial shortening). In the Subgroup .2 the fracture line is oblique and slopes upwards and backwards and the displacement is posterior (or dorsal). In the Subgroup .3 the fracture line is oblique and slopes upwards and forwards and the displacement is anterior (or volar).

The **subgroups of A3,** the extra-articular multifragmentary fractures, are classified according to the degree of fragmentation and compression of the metaphysis.

Fig. 53   **Radius/Ulna distal: the subgroups and their qualifications**

A1   Extra-articular fracture, of the ulna, radius intact
  .1   styloid process
  .2   metaphyseal simple
  .3   metaphyseal multifragmentary
              1) wedge   *2) complex*

A2   Extra-articular fracture, of the radius, simple and impacted
              1) radio-ulnar dislocation (= fracture of styloid process)
              2) simple fracture of ulnar neck   3) multifragmentary fracture of ulnar neck
              4) fracture of ulnar head   5) fracture of ulnar head and neck
              6) fracture of the ulna proximal to the neck
  .1   without any tilt
  .2   with dorsal tilt (Pouteau-Colles)
  .3   with volar tilt (Goyrand-Smith)

A3   Extra-articular fracture, of the radius, multifragmentary
              1) radio-ulnar dislocation (= fracture of styloid process)
              2) simple fracture of ulnar neck   3) multifragmentary fracture of ulnar neck
              4) fracture of ulnar head   5) fracture of ulnar head and neck
              6) fracture of the ulna proximal to the neck
  .1   impacted with axial shortening
  .2   with a wedge
  .3   complex

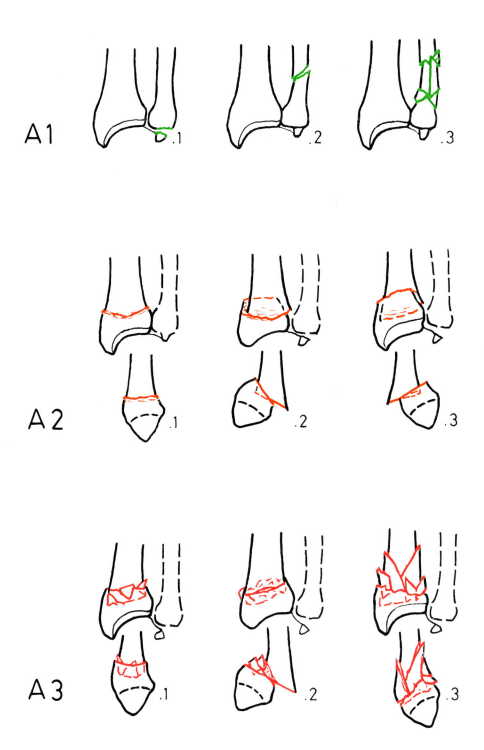

A1

   .1   .2   .3

A2

   .1   .2   .3

A3

   .1   .2   .3

The **subgroups of B1**, the partial articular fractures in the sagittal plane, are classified according to the state and location of the articular wedge fragment. The fracture belongs to Subgroup .1 if the wedge is intact and lateral, to the Subgroup .2 if the lateral wedge is fragmented, and to the Subgroup .3 if the wedge is medial (the surgical approach is more difficult for medial wedges).

The **subgroups of B2**, the partial articular fractures in the frontal plane involving the dorsal rim, are classified according to the number of articular fragments and the degree of dorsal displacement.

The **subgroups of B3**, the partial articular fractures in the frontal plane involving the volar rim (reverse Barton, Goyrand-Smith II), are classified according to the size and number of the volar rim fragments.

Fig. 54   **B1   Partial articular fracture, of the radius, sagittal**
1) radio-ulnar dislocation (= f. styloid process)
2) simple fracture of ulnar neck   3) multifragmentary fracture of ulnar neck
4) fracture of ulnar head   5) fracture of ulnar head and neck
6) fracture of the ulna proximal to the neck
.1   lateral simple
.2   lateral multifragmentary
.3   medial

B2   Partial articular fracture, of the radius, dorsal rim (Barton)
1) radio-ulnar dislocation (= f. styloid process)
2) simple fracture of ulnar neck   3) multifragmentary fracture of ulnar neck
4) fracture of ulnar head   5) fracture of ulnar head and neck
6) fracture of the ulna proximal to the neck
.1   simple
.2   with lateral sagittal fracture
.3   with dorsal dislocation of the carpus

B3   Partial articular fracture, of the radius, volar rim (reverse Barton, Goyrand-Smith II)
1) radio-ulnar dislocation (= f. styloid process)
2) simple fracture of ulnar neck   3) multifragmentary fracture of ulnar neck
4) fracture of ulnar head   5) fracture of ulnar head and neck
6) fracture of the ulna proximal to the neck
.1   simple, with a small fragment
.2   simple, with a large fragment
.3   multifragmentary

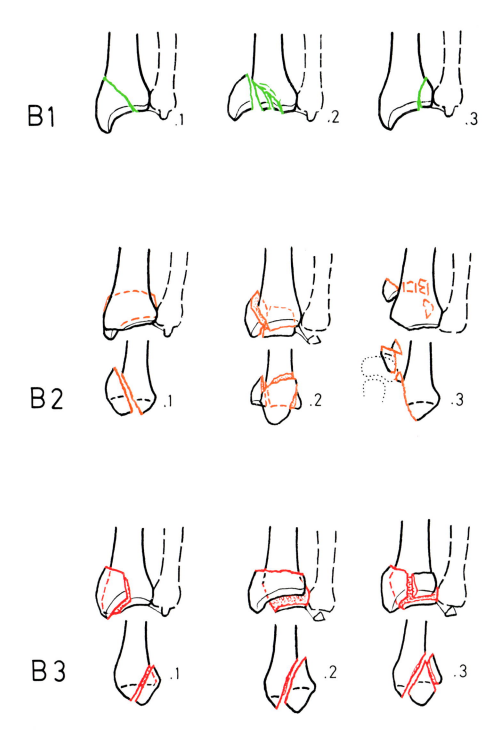

B1

  .1   .2   .3

B2

  .1   .2   .3

B3

  .1   .2   .3

The **subgroups of C1**, the complete articular fractures of the radius with simple articular and simple metaphyseal components, are classified according to the direction of the articular fracture plane. The fractures in the sagittal plane are surgically more accessible than the fractures in the frontal plane.

The **subgroups of C2**, the complete articular fractures of the radius with simple articular and multifragmentary metaphyseal components, are classified according to the direction of the articular fracture plane and the degree of metaphyseal fragmentation.

The **subgroups of C3**, the complete articular multifragmentary fractures of the radius, are classified according to the extent of the metaphyseal fragmentation. The articular fracture is always multifragmentary.

Fig. 55   **C1**   **Complete articular fracture, of the radius, articular simple, metaphyseal simple**
> *1) radio-ulnar dislocation (= f. styloid process)*
> *2) simple fracture of ulnar neck   3) multifragmentary fracture of ulnar neck*
> *4) fracture of ulnar head   5) fracture of ulnar head and neck*
> *6) fracture of the ulna proximal to the neck*

     .1   postero-medial articular fragment
     .2   sagittal articular fracture line
     .3   frontal articular fracture line

   C2   **Complete articular fracture, of the radius, articular simple, metaphyseal multifragmentary**
> *1) radio-ulnar dislocation (= f. styloid process)*
> *2) simple fracture of ulnar neck   3) multifragmentary fracture of ulnar neck*
> *4) fracture of ulnar head   5) fracture of ulnar head and neck*
> *6) fracture of the ulna proximal to the neck*

     .1   sagittal articular fracture line
     .2   frontal articular fracture line
     .3   extending into the diaphysis

   C3   **Complete articular fracture, of the radius, multifragmentary**
> *1) radio-ulnar dislocation (= f. styloid process)*
> *2) simple fracture of ulnar neck   3) multifragmentary fracture of ulnar neck*
> *4) fracture of ulnar head   5) fracture of ulnar head and neck*
> *6) fracture of the ulna proximal to the neck*

     .1   metaphyseal simple
     .2   metaphyseal multifragmentary
     .3   extending into the diaphysis

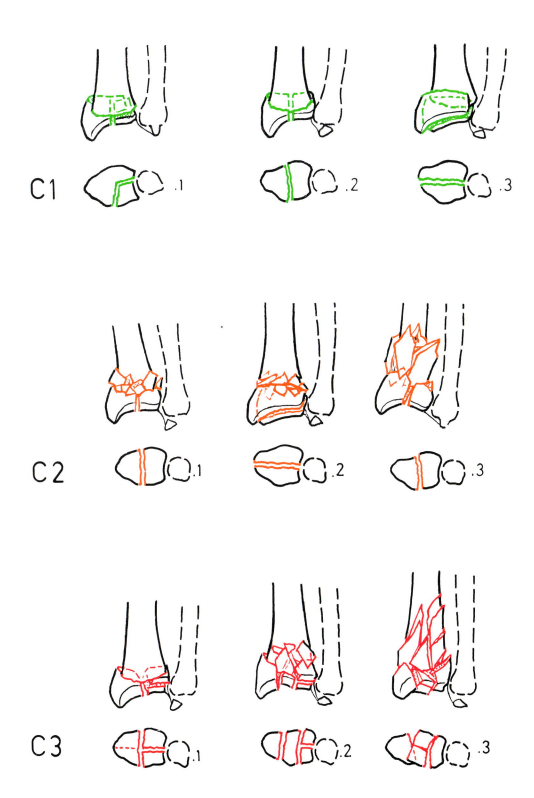

C1

.1

.2

.3

C2

.1

.2

.3

C3

.1

.2

.3

115

3. Femur = 3

3.1 Femur, Proximal Segment = 31-

3.1.1 The Types

The proximal segment is defined by a line passing transversely through the lower edge of the lesser trochanter. We distinguish three fracture types according to the three topographical areas of this segment: the trochanteric area, the neck and the head.

The trochanteric area is delimited by the intertrochanteric line above and the distal limit of the proximal segment below. All fractures in this area are considered as trochanteric fractures. The head is defined as that portion of the proximal segment covered by articular cartilage.

Please note: In the proximal segment, *isolated avulsions of the greater and lesser trochanter* are classified in 31-D1, as is the case for any unclassifiable fracture

---

Fig. 56   **Femur proximal: the bone, the segment, and the types**

3   Femur
31-   Femur proximal
31A-   Femur proximal, trochanteric area fracture
31B-   Femur proximal, neck fracture
31C-   Femur proximal, head fracture

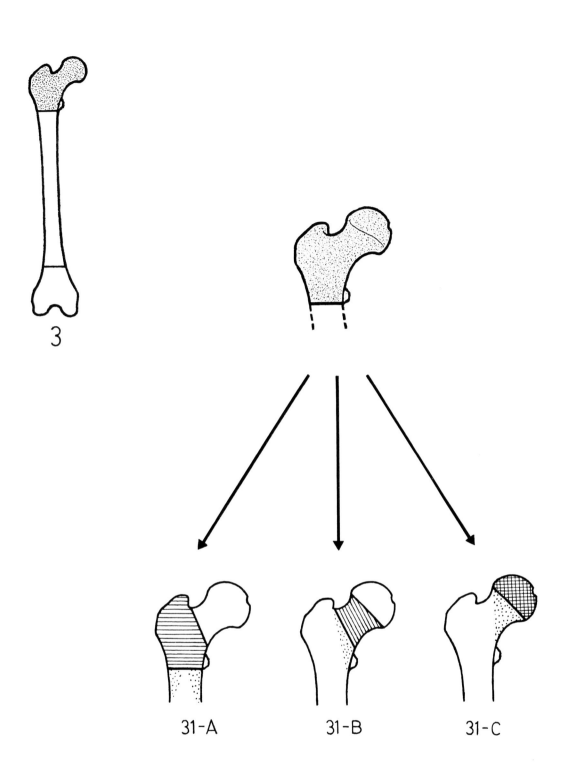

3

31-A   31-B   31-C

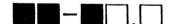

3.1.2 The Groups

Type A fractures are the fractures of the **trochanteric area**. These are divided into three groups:

Group **A1** are the simple pertrochanteric fractures. In these the fracture line can begin anywhere on the greater trochanter and end either above or below the lesser trochanter. There are only two fragments and the medial cortex is interrupted in only one place.

Group **A2** are the multifragmentary pertrochanteric fractures. The fracture line can start laterally anywhere on the greater trochanter and runs towards the medial cortex which is broken in two different places. This results in the detachment of a third fragment which includes the lesser trochanter.

Group **A3** are the intertrochanteric fractures. In these the fracture line passes between the two trochanters above the lesser trochanter medially and below the crest of the vastus lateralis laterally. To be classified as "intertrochanteric", the fracture must have its center above the transverse line which delineates the inferior limit of the trochanteric area. If the center is below this line, the fracture is considered as subtrochanteric.

Type B, the neck fractures are divided into three groups: **B1** are the subcapital fractures with slight displacement, **B2** are the transcervical fractures and **B3** are the subcapital fractures with significant displacement.

Type C, the head fractures, are divided into three groups. The Group **C1** is comprised of split fractures, the Group **C2** of depression fractures, and the Group **C3** of the combined head and neck fractures.

Fig. 57   **Femur proximal: the groups**

A1	Trochanteric area fracture, pertrochanteric simple
A2	Trochanteric area fracture, pertrochanteric multifragmentary
A3	Trochanteric area fracture, intertrochanteric
B1	Neck fracture, subcapital, with slight displacement
B2	Neck fracture, transcervical
B3	Neck fracture, subcapital, with marked displacement
C1	Head fracture, split
C2	Head fracture, with depression
C3	Head fracture, with neck fracture

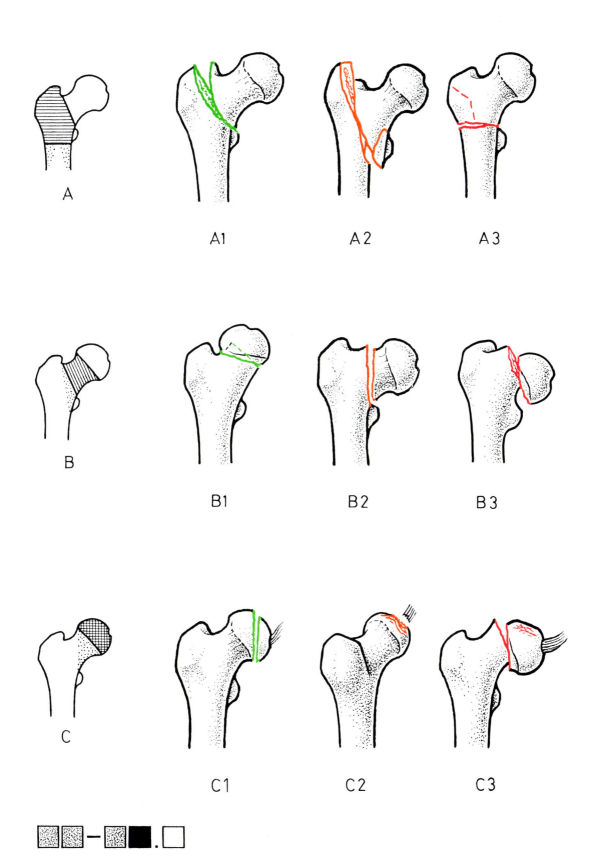

A

A1   A2   A3

B

B1   B2   B3

C

C1   C2   C3

119

3.1.3   The Subgroups and Their Qualifications

The **subgroups of A1**, the simple pertrochanteric fractures, are as follows: The subgroup .1 includes the pertrochanteric fractures whose fracture line follows the intertrochanteric line. The subgroup .2 includes the simple fractures whose line begins anywhere on the greater trochanter laterally and ends in the medial cortex just above the upper limit of the lesser trochanter. Generally the fractures in the subgroup .2 show some varus displacement and, unlike the subgroup .1, may be impacted medially. The subgroup .3 includes the pertrochanteric fractures whose fracture line starts anywhere on the greater trochanter laterally and ends either at the lower limit of the lesser trochanter (1) or in the medial cortex of the diaphysis below the lesser trochanter (2).

The **subgroups of A2**, the multifragmentary pertrochanteric fractures, are classified according to the number and extent of the intermediate fragments. They always have a posteromedial fragment which is comprised of the lesser trochanter and the adjacent medial cortex. In the subgroup .1, there is only one intermediate fragment; in the subgroups .2 and .3 there are several. In the subgroup .3 the lower extent of the fracture is far below the lesser trochanter (at least more than 1 cm).

The **subgroups of A3**, the intertrochanteric fractures, are classified according to the pattern of the fracture line. The subgroup .1 includes the simple oblique intertrochanteric fractures (the so-called reverse intertrochanteric fractures). The subgroup .2 includes the simple transverse intertrochanteric fractures. The subgroup .3 includes the multifragmentary intertrochanteric fractures which always have a detached medial cortical fragment. Any one of these three subgroups may be associated with cracks in the greater trochanter.

Fig. 58   **Femur proximal: the subgroups and their qualifications**

A 1   Trochanteric area fracture, pertrochanteric simple
    .1   along the intertrochanteric line
    .2   through the greater trochanter
              1) non-impacted   *2) impacted*
    .3   below the lesser trochanter
              1) high variety   *2) low variety*
A 2   Trochanteric area fracture, pertrochanteric multifragmentary
    .1   with one intermediate fragment
    .2   with several intermediate fragments
    .3   extending more than 1 cm below the lesser trochanter
A 3   Trochanteric area fracture, intertrochanteric
    .1   simple, oblique
    .2   simple, transverse
    .3   multifragmentary
              1) extending to the greater trochanter
              2) extending to the neck

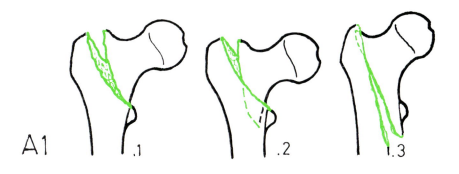

A1

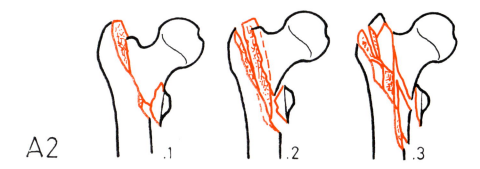

A2

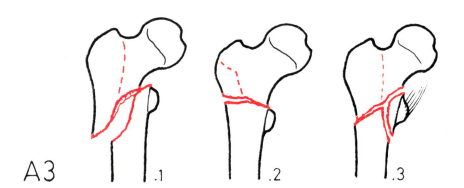

A3

121

In the **subgroups of B1**, the subcapital fractures with little or no displacement, the contact between the head and the neck is always maintained. These subgroups are as follows: subgroup .1 includes fractures in which the head is impacted in marked valgus (Garden 1/1). The subgroup .2 comprises fractures in which the head is impacted in mild valgus (Garden 1/2). The subgroup .3 is made up of fractures with no displacement (Garden II). The subgroups .1 and .2 can be further divided according to the degree of posterior tilting of the femoral head.

In the **subgroups of B2**, the transcervical fractures, the proximal end of the fracture line begins at some distance from the head. These subgroups are as follows: The subgroup .1 includes basicervical fractures. The subgroup .2 are the midcervical fractures with a varus displacement. They are the result of an adduction injury. The subgroup .3 are the midcervical fractures which are caused by a vertical shear.

In the **subgroups of B3**, the displaced subcapital fractures with a poor prognosis, the fracture line originates proximally always at the border of the articular cartilage. These subgroups are as follows: The subgroup .1 includes fractures with mild varus displacement (Garden III/1), the subgroup .2 fractures with mild vertical translation (Garden IV/1), and subgroup .3, the fractures with significant varus displacement (Garden III/2) or vertical translation (Garden IV/2).

Fig. 59   **B1**   **Neck fracture, subcapital, with slight displacement**
       .1   impacted in valgus ≥15°
            1) posterior tilt <15°   *2) posterior tilt >15°*
       .2   impacted in valgus <15°
            1) posterior tilt <15°   *2) posterior tilt >15°*
       .3   non-impacted

       B2   **Neck fracture, transcervical**
       .1   basicervical
       .2   midcervical adduction
       .3   midcervical shear

       B3   **Neck fracture, subcapital, non-impacted, displaced**
       .1   moderate displacement in varus and external rotation
       .2   moderate displacement with vertical translation and external rotation
       .3   marked displacement
            1) in varus   *2) with translation*

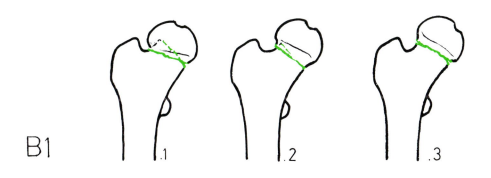

B1   .1   .2   .3

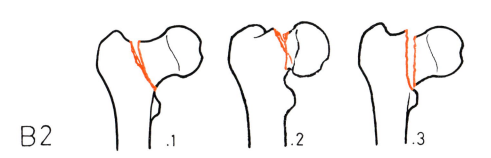

B2   .1   .2   .3

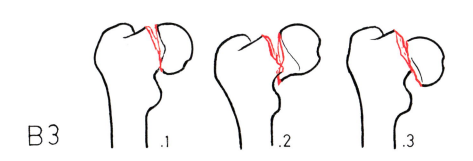

B3   .1   .2   .3

The **subgroups of C1, C2** and **C3** are rare. They are almost always associated with a traumatic postero-superior dislocation of the hip.

Fig. 60   **C 1**   **Head fracture, split**
         .1   avulsion of the ligamentum teres
         .2   with rupture of the ligamentum teres
         .3   large fragment

         C 2   **Head fracture, with depression**
         .1   posterior and superior
         .2   anterior and superior
         .3   split-depression

         C 3   **Head fracture, with neck fracture**
         .1   split and transcervical neck fracture
         .2   split and subcapital neck fracture
         .3   depression and neck fracture

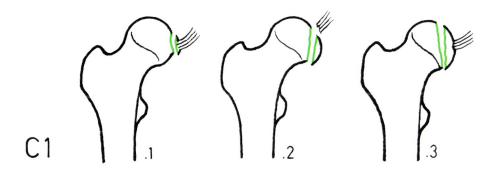

C1   .1   .2   .3

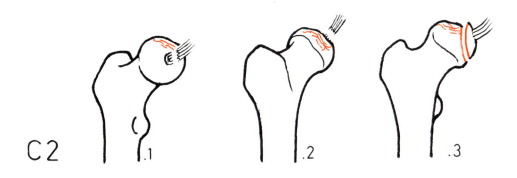

C2   .1   .2   .3

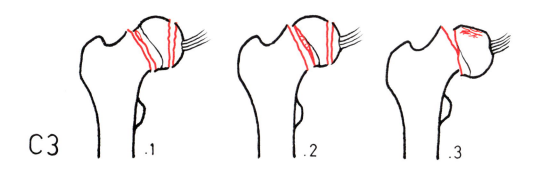

C3   .1   .2   .3

3.1.4   Comments about Fractures of the Proximal Femur

1) The surgical limit between the trochanteric area and the diaphysial segment is a transverse line through the lower limit of the lesser trochanter.

Fractures with lines beginning distally in the shaft and ending proximally above the lesser trochanter are designated as ***intertrochanteric*** if their center is located above the distal limit of the trochanteric area (transverse line passing through the distal limit of the lesser trochanter), and as ***subtrochanteric*** diaphyseal fractures if the center is below this limit, but above a point 3 cm below the distal limit of the lesser trochanter.

2) The classification of femoral neck fractures now most widely in use was proposed by *Garden* (1964, 1966). Garden's classification, however, deals only with subcapital fractures and makes no reference to transcervical fractures. The four stages in the Garden classification depend on the direction of the stress trabeculae within the femoral head and neck (see Fig. 61). In Garden's stage I the head is displaced into valgus and impacted. In stage II, there is no displacement of the head. In stage III, the head is displaced into varus, and in stage IV, the rupture of all synovial and capsular attachments results in an upward and outward translation of the neck in relation to the head.

If one considers the prognosis there is a clear separation between Garden I and II, on the one hand, and Garden III and IV, on the other. This discrepancy has led us to classify Garden I and II in B1 and Garden III and IV in B3 and to assign the transcervical fractures which have an intermediate prognosis into B2.

Fig. 61   **The *Garden* Classification of neck fractures (1964)**

Garden I   Incomplete fracture. The medial group of trabeculae in the femoral neck shows a "greenstick" fracture in a valgus position.

Garden II   Complete fracture without displacement. The line of the medial trabecular group is undisturbed.

Garden III   Complete fracture with partial displacement. The capital fragment is tilted into a varus position, and its medial trabeculae are out of line with their fellows in the pelvis.

Garden IV   Complete fracture with full displacement. The capital fragment has returned to its normal position in the acetabulum, and its medial trabeculae are in line with their pelvic projections.

126

Garden 1964

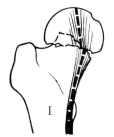
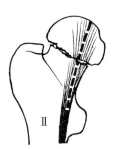
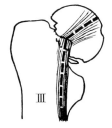
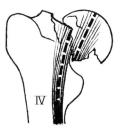

3.2   Femur, Diaphyseal Segment = 32-

3.2.1   The Types

The proximal limit of the diaphyseal segment is a transverse line passing through the inferior edge of the lesser trochanter.

Fig. 62   **Femur diaphysis: the segment, the types**

32-   Femur diaphysis
32-A   Femur diaphysis, simple fracture
32-B   Femur diaphysis, wedge fracture
32-C   Femur diaphysis, complex fracture

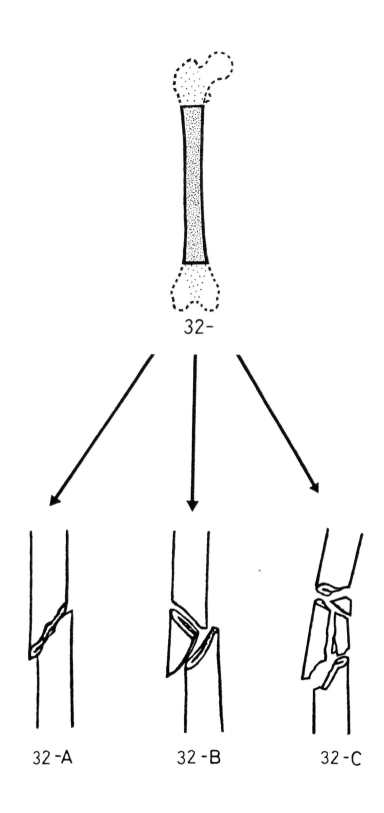

32-

32-A   32-B   32-C

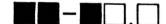

3.2.2   The Groups

Fig. 63   **Femur diaphysis: the groups**

A1   Simple fracture, spiral
A2   Simple fracture, oblique ($\geq 30°$)
A3   Simple fracture, transverse ($< 30°$)

B1   Wedge fracture, spiral wedge
B2   Wedge fracture, bending wedge
B3   Wedge fracture, fragmented wedge

C1   Complex fracture, spiral
C2   Complex fracture, segmental
C3   Complex fracture, irregular

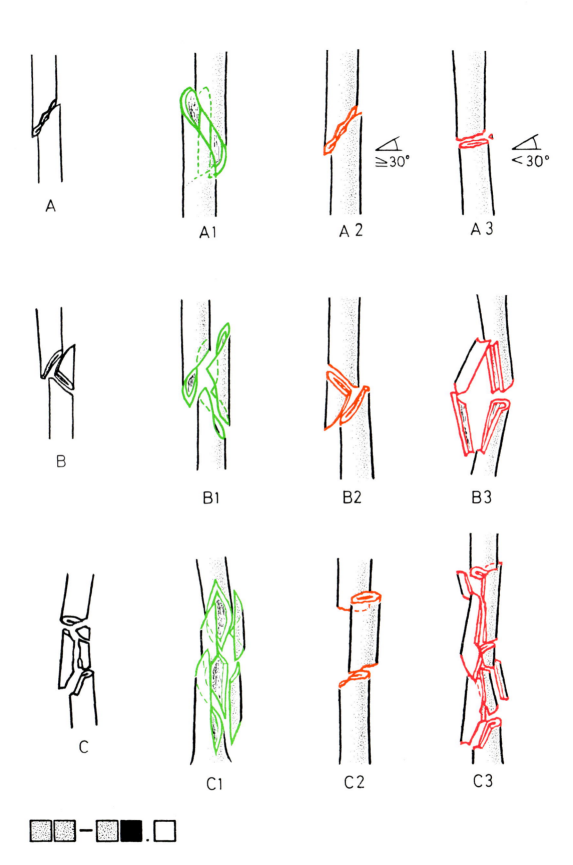

A

A1

A2   ≧30°

A3   <30°

B

B1

B2

B3

C

C1

C2

C3

131

3.2.3   The Subgroups and Their Qualifications

Fig. 64   **Femur diaphysis: the subgroups and their qualifications**

A 1   Simple fracture, spiral
.1   subtrochanteric zone
.2   middle zone
.3   distal zone

A 2   Simple fracture, oblique (≥30°)
.1   subtrochanteric zone
.2   middle zone
.3   distal zone

A 3   Simple fracture, transverse (<30°)
.1   subtrochanteric zone
.2   middle zone
.3   distal zone

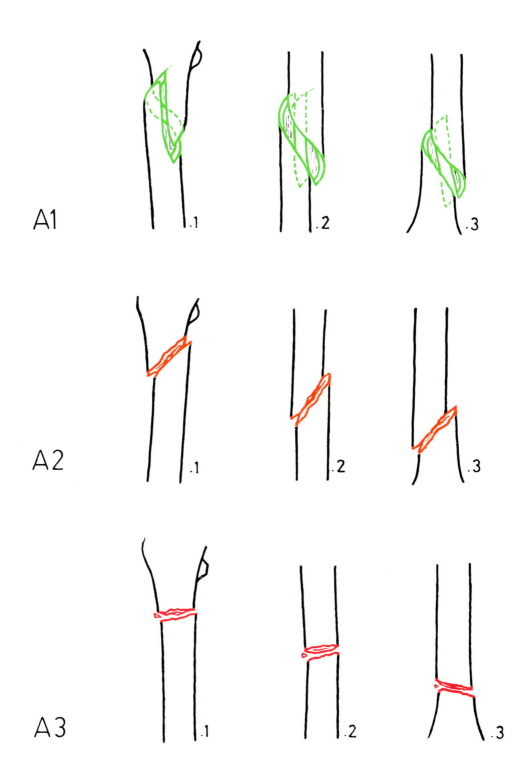

A1

.1   .2   .3

A2

.1   .2   .3

A3

.1   .2   .3

Femur, Diaphysis = 32- (Cont.)

Fig. 65   **B1**   **Wedge fracture, spiral wedge**
                    .1   subtrochanteric zone
                    .2   middle zone
                    .3   distal zone

             B2   **Wedge fracture, bending wedge**
                    .1   subtrochanteric zone
                    .2   middle zone
                    .3   distal zone

             B3   **Wedge fracture, fragmented wedge**
                              1) spiral wedge   *2) bending wedge*
                    .1   subtrochanteric zone
                    .2   middle zone
                    .3   distal zone

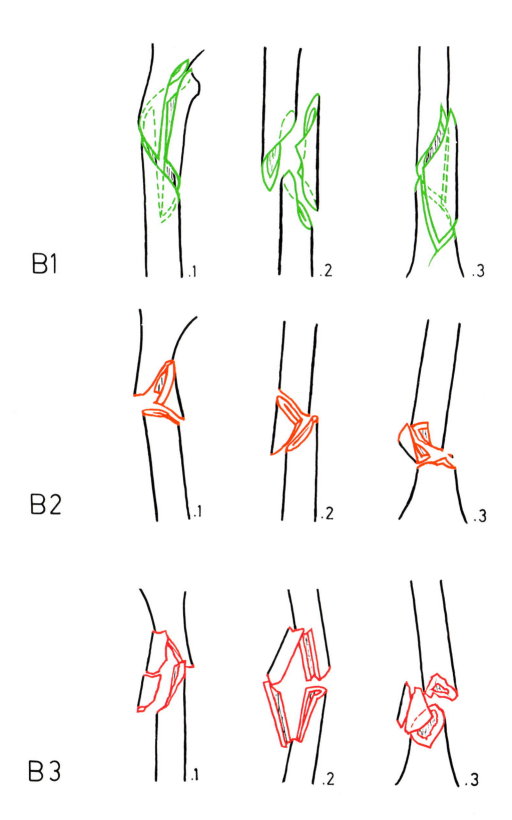

B1 .1 .2 .3

B2 .1 .2 .3

B3 .1 .2 .3

135

Fig. 66   **C1**   **Complex fracture, spiral**
                        1) pure diaphyseal   *2) proximal diaphysio-metaphyseal*
                        3) distal diaphysio-metaphyseal
            .1   with two intermediate fragments
            .2   with three intermediate fragments
            .3   with more than three intermediate fragments

            C2   **Complex fracture, segmental**
            .1   with one intermediate segmental fragment
                        1) pure diaphyseal   *2) proximal diaphysio-metaphyseal*
                        3) distal diaphysio-metaphyseal   *4) oblique lines*
                        5) transverse and oblique lines
            .2   with one intermediate segmental and additional wedge fragment(s)
                        1) pure diaphyseal   *2) proximal diaphysio-metaphyseal*
                        3) distal diaphysio-metaphyseal   *4) distal wedge*
                        5) two wedges, proximal and distal
            .3   with two intermediate segmental fragments
                        1) pure diaphyseal   *2) proximal diaphysio-metaphyseal*
                        3) distal diaphysio-metaphyseal

            C3   **Complex fracture, irregular**
            .1   with two or three intermediate fragments
                        1) two main intermediate fragments
                        2) three main intermediate fragments
            .2   with limited shattering (< 5 cm)
                        1) proximal zone   *2) middle zone*   *3) distal zone*
            .3   with extensive shattering (≥ 5 cm)
                        1) pure diaphyseal   *2) proximal diaphysio-metaphyseal*
                        3) distal diaphysio-metaphyseal

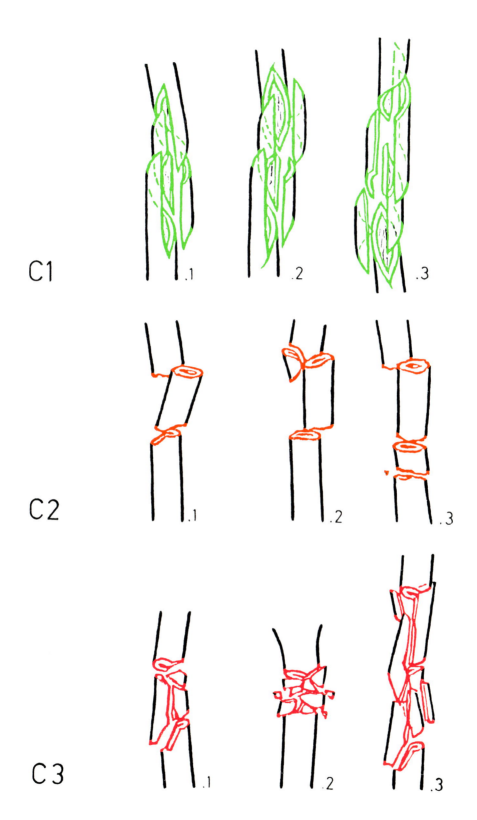

C1

.1 .2 .3

C2

.1 .2 .3

C3

.1 .2 .3

137

3.3   Femur, Distal Segment = 33-

3.3.1   The Types

The proximal limit of the distal segment is determined by the square method where the side of the square is the same length as the widest part of the epiphysis. The three fracture types in this segment are **A**: extra-articular, **B**: partial articular, and **C**: complete articular fractures.

Fig. 67   **Femur distal: the bone, the segment, and the types**

3   Femur
33-   Femur distal
33-A   Femur distal, extra-articular fracture
33-B   Femur distal, partial articular fracture
33-C   Femur distal, complete articular fracture

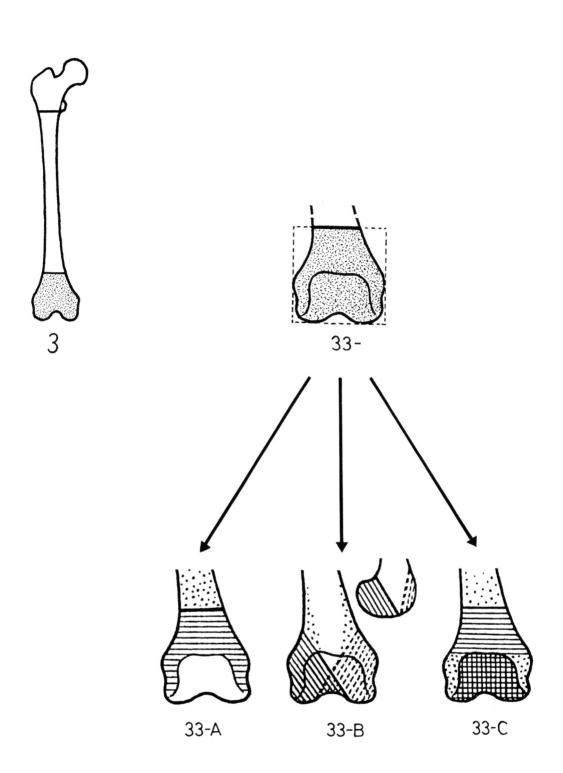

3

33-

33-A   33-B   33-C

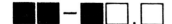

3.3.2   The Groups

The Type A fractures are divided into three groups of increasing severity. **Group A1** are the simple extra-articular fractures. **Group A2** are the metaphyseal wedge fractures, and **Group A3** are the metaphyseal complex fractures.

The Type B fractures, i.e. partial articular fractures, are classified according to the plane of the fracture and the direction of the fracture line. **B1** are the lateral sagittal fractures with the fracture line running upwards and outwards and detaching the lateral condyle. **B2** includes the medial sagittal fractures with the fracture line running oblique upwards and inwards and detaching the medial condyle. **B3** are the fractures in the frontal plane.

The Type C fractures, i.e. complete articular fractures, are classified according to the pattern of the articular and metaphyseal components. **C1** are the simple articular and simple metaphyseal fractures. **C2** includes the simple articular and multifragmentary metaphyseal fractures, and **C3** are the multifragmentary articular fractures . The morphology of the metaphyseal component is not important in defining the group.

Fig. 68   **Femur distal: the groups**

A1   Extra-articular fracture, simple
A2   Extra-articular fracture, metaphyseal wedge
A3   Extra-articular fracture, metaphyseal complex

B1   Partial articular fracture, lateral condyle, sagittal
B2   Partial articular fracture, medial condyle, sagittal
B3   Partial articular fracture, frontal

C1   Complete articular fracture, articular simple, metaphyseal simple
C2   Complete articular fracture, articular simple, metaphyseal multifragmentary
C3   Complete articular fracture multifragmentary

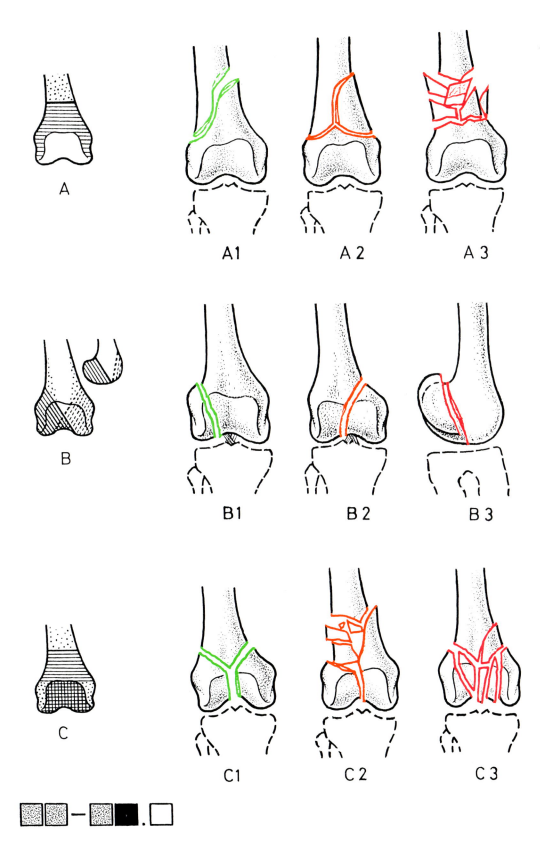

A

A1 A2 A3

B

B1 B2 B3

C

C1 C2 C3

3.3.3   The Subgroups and Their Qualifications

The **subgroups of A1**, the simple extra-articular fractures, are as follows:
The subgroup .1 includes the epicondylar avulsions of the collateral ligaments. Subgroups .2 and .3 are distinguished according to the direction of the fracture line. Thus in subgroup .2 the fracture line is oblique or spiral, and in subgroup .3 it is transverse.

The **subgroups of A2**, the extra-articular wedge fractures, are classified according to the location and the state of the wedge. In the subgroup .1 the wedge is in one piece. In the subgroup .2 it is lateral and fragmented. In subgroup .3 it is medial and fragmented.

The **subgroups of A3**, the metaphyseal complex fractures, are classified according to the number and extent of the fragments.

Fig. 69   **Femur distal: the subgroups and their qualifications**

A1   Extra-articular fracture, simple
     .1   apophyseal
            1) avulsion of the lateral epicondyle
            2) avulsion of the medial epicondyle
     .2   metaphyseal oblique or spiral
     .3   metaphyseal transverse

A2   Extra-articular fracture, metaphyseal wedge
     .1   intact
            1) lateral   *2) medial*
     .2   fragmented, lateral
     .3   fragmented, medial

A3   Extra-articular fracture, metaphyseal complex
     .1   with an intermediate split segment
     .2   irregular, limited to the metaphysis
     .3   irregular, extending into the diaphysis

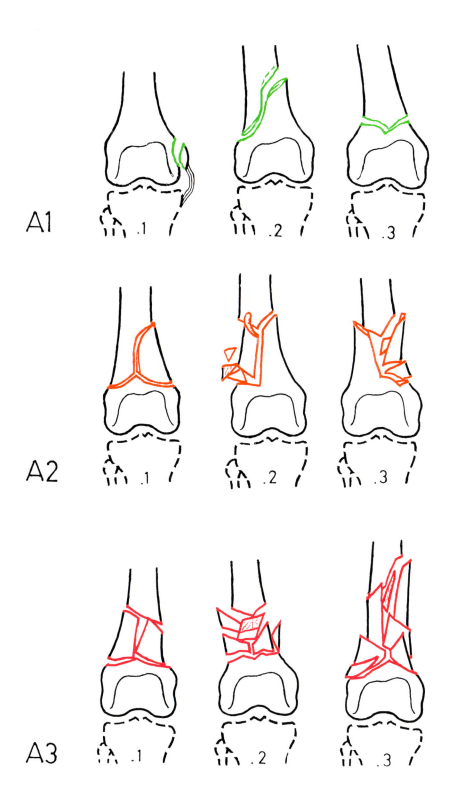

A1

.1   .2   .3

A2

.1   .2   .3

A3

.1   .2   .3

The **subgroups of B1, B2,** and **B3** fractures are as follows:

Since the prognosis is better and the surgical approach is easier for the lateral sagittal condylar fractures, they are classified as B1 and the medial as B2. In both B1 and B2, the subgroups .2 and .3 are fractures which involve the weight bearing surface. The fractures in the frontal plane, the most difficult to treat, are classified as B3.

Fig. 70   **B1   Partial articular fracture, lateral condyle, sagittal**
.1   simple, through the notch
.2   simple, through the load-bearing surface
.3   multifragmentary

B2   Partial articular fracture, medial condyle, sagittal
.1   simple, through the notch
.2   simple, through the load-bearing surface
.3   multifragmentary

B3   Partial articular fracture, frontal
.1   anterior and lateral flake fracture
.2   unicondylar posterior (Hoffa)
1) lateral   *2) medial*
.3   bicondylar posterior

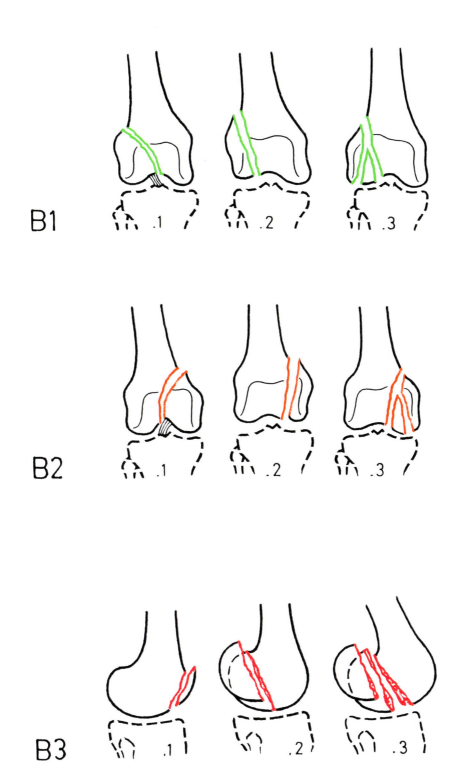

B1   .1   .2   .3

B2   .1   .2   .3

B3   .1   .2   .3

The **subgroups of C1, C2,** and **C3** fractures, i.e. complete articular fractures, are as follows:

The subgroups of **C1** fractures are classified according to the pattern of the fracture and the degree of displacement. The subgroups of **C2** are classified according to the location and fragmentation of the metaphyseal wedge fragment. In C2.1 the wedge is intact. Further subdivision is based on whether the wedge is lateral or medial; this is coded as a qualification of the subgroup. Thus C2.1(1) represents the lateral wedge and C2.1(2) the medial. In C2.2 the wedge is fragmented. This subgroup is further subdivided on the basis of the wedge being medial or lateral. Thus C2.2(1) represents a lateral wedge and C2.2(2) the medial. In C2.3 the metaphyseal fracture is complex. The subgroups of C3 fractures, the multifragmentary complete articular fractures, are classified according to the number of intermediate articular fragments and the extent of the metaphyseal fragmentation.

Fig. 71
C 1   Complete articular fracture, articular simple, metaphyseal simple
.1   T- or Y-shaped, with slight displacement
.2   T- or Y-shaped, with marked displacement
.3   T-shaped epiphyseal

C 2   Complete articular fracture, articular simple, metaphyseal multifragmentary
.1   with an intact wedge
            1) lateral   *2) medial*
.2   with a fragmented wedge
            1) lateral   *2) medial*
.3   complex

C 3   Complete articular fracture, multifragmentary
.1   metaphyseal simple
.2   metaphyseal multifragmentary
.3   metaphysio-diaphyseal multifragmentary

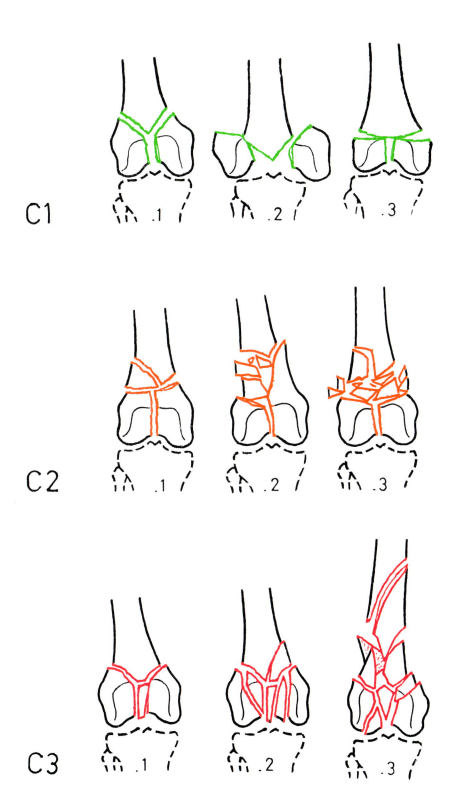

C1 .1 .2 .3

C2 .1 .2 .3

C3 .1 .2 .3

147

4. Tibia/Fibula = 4

4.1 Tibia/Fibula, Proximal Segment = 41-

4.1.1 The Types

This segment is defined by the square method (see pages 10 and 11). Three fracture types can be distinguished as follows: The extra-articular **Type A** fractures, the partial articular **Type B** fractures in which only one part of the proximal articular surface of the tibia is separated from the diaphysis, and the complete articular **Type C** fractures in which the proximal articular surface is divided into at least two fragments and which themselves are completely detached from the diaphysis.

The Type B and Type C lesions fit under the heading of "tibial plateau" fractures.

Fig. 72   **Tibia/Fibula proximal: the bone, the segment, and the types**

4   Tibia/Fibula
41-   Tibia/Fibula proximal
41-A   Tibia/Fibula proximal, extra-articular fracture
41-B   Tibia/Fibula proximal, partial articular fracture
41-C   Tibia/Fibula proximal, complete articular fracture

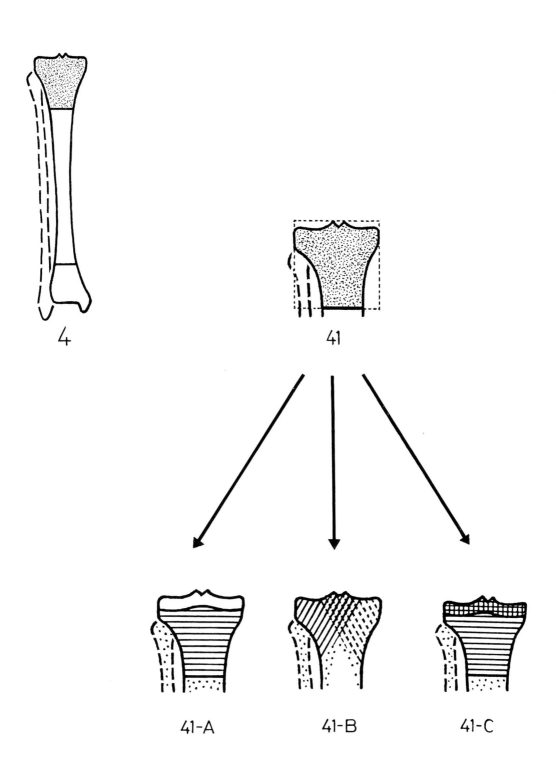

4

41

41-A   41-B   41-C

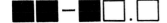

4.1.2   The Groups

The Type A fractures, are divided into the following groups: The **Group A1** includes the more frequent extra-articular avulsion fractures involving the major ligaments of the knee joint , the **Group A2** includes the metaphyseal simple fractures, and the **Group A3** includes the metaphyseal multifragmentary fractures.

The Type B fractures, i.e. the partial articular fractures, are classified on the basis of the severity of the articular lesion which depends on whether it is an isolated split or an isolated depression of the articular surface or an association of a split with a depression. Thus, arranged in an ascending order of severity, the **Group B1** includes only the pure split fractures, the **Group B2** includes the depression fractures, and the **Group B3** includes the association of a split with a depression of the articular surface.

The Type C fractures, i.e. the complete articular fractures, are classified according to the pattern of the articular and metaphyseal components. **C1** includes the simple articular and simple metaphyseal fractures. **C2** includes the simple articular and multifragmentary metaphyseal fractures. **C3** includes the multifragmentary articular fractures regardless of the pattern of the metaphyseal component.

Fig. 73   **Tibia/Fibula proximal: the groups**

A1   Extra-articular fracture, avulsion
A2   Extra-articular fracture, metaphyseal simple
A3   Extra-articular fracture, metaphyseal multifragmentary

B1   Partial articular fracture, pure split
B2   Partial articular fracture, pure depression
B3   Partial articular fracture, split-depression

C1   Complete articular fracture, articular simple, metaphyseal simple
C2   Complete articular fracture, articular simple, metaphyseal multifragmentary
C3   Complete articular fracture, multifragmentary

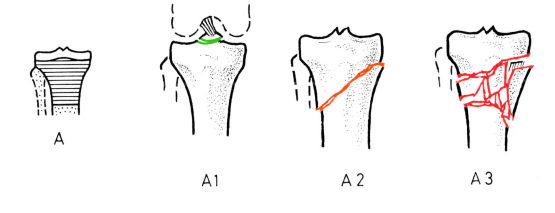

A   A1   A 2   A 3

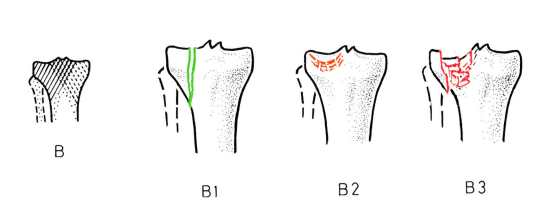

B   B1   B 2   B 3

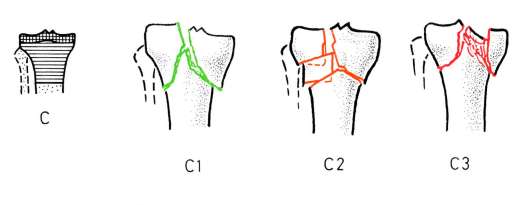

C   C1   C 2   C3

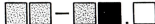

4.1.3   The Subgroups and Their Qualifications

The **subgroups of** the **Group A1** fractures are a mixture. Only the subgroup A1.2, the avulsion of the tibial tubercle, is a true extra-articular fracture. The other two subgroups are included because of their high frequency. Subgroup A1.1 is the avulsion of the styloid process of the fibula, and subgroup A1.3 is the avulsion of the insertion of either the anterior or posterior cruciate ligament.

The **subgroups of** the **Group A2**, the simple metaphyseal fractures, are classified according to the direction of the fracture line. The oblique fractures in the frontal plane are the simplest and thus are classified in the subgroup A2.1. The oblique fractures in the sagittal plane have a high risk of vascular damage related to their displacement and are thus classified in the subgroup A2.2. The transverse fractures, classified in the subgroup A2.3, are the most difficult to treat and their prognosis is usually poorer than in the previous subgroups.

The **subgroups of** the **Group A3**, the multifragmentary metaphyseal fractures, are classified according to the number and extent of the intermediary fragments. The subgroup A3.1 includes the fractures with an intact wedge, the subgroup A3.2 the fractures with a fragmented wedge, and the subgroup A3.3 the complex metaphyseal fractures.

Fig. 74   **Tibia/Fibula proximal: the subgroups and their qualifications**

A 1   Extra-articular fracture, avulsion
- .1   of the fibular head
- .2   of the tibial tuberosity
- .3   of the cruciate insertion
  - *1) anterior*   *2) posterior*

A 2   Extra-articular fracture, metaphyseal simple
- .1   oblique in the frontal plane
- .2   oblique in the sagittal plane
- .3   transverse

A 3   Extra-articular fracture, metaphyseal multifragmentary
- .1   intact wedge
  - *1) lateral*   *2) medial*
- .2   fragmented wedge
  - *1) lateral*   *2) medial*
- .3   complex
  - *1) slightly displaced*   *2) significantly displaced*

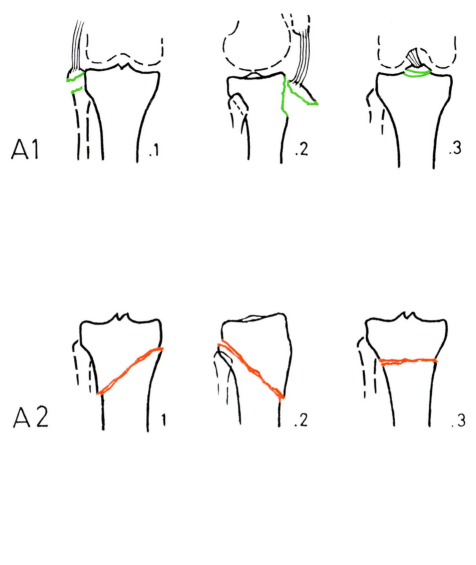

A1   .1   .2   .3

A2   1   .2   .3

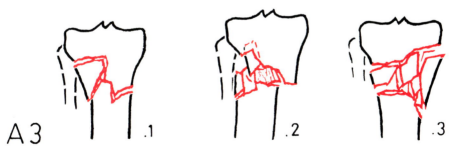

A3   .1   .2   .3

The classification of the **subgroups of the Type B**, the partial articular fractures, depends mainly on whether the fracture involves the lateral or the medial articular surface of the proximal tibia. The prognosis is poorer for the medial fractures, which explains why they are classified after the lateral ones.

The occasional disruption of the contralateral ligament is indicated by qualification 5) and disruption of the cruciate ligament is denoted as 6).

Fig. 75   **B1**   **Partial articular fracture, pure split**
.1   of the lateral surface
  1) marginal   2) sagittal   3) frontal anterior   4) frontal posterior
.2   of the medial surface
  1) marginal   2) sagittal   3) frontal anterior   4) frontal posterior
.3   oblique, involving the tibial spines and one of the surfaces
  1) lateral   2) medial

B2   **Partial articular fracture, pure depression**
.1   lateral total
  1) one piece depression   2) mosaic-like depression
.2   lateral limited
  1) peripheral   2) central   3) anterior   4) posterior
.3   medial
  1) central 2) anterior   3) posterior   4) total

B3   **Partial articular fracture, split-depression**
.1   lateral
  1) antero-lateral depression   2) postero-lateral depression
  3) antero-medial depression   4) postero-medial depression
.2   medial
  1) antero-lateral depression   2) postero-lateral depression
  3) antero-medial depression   4) postero-medial depression
.3   oblique, involving the tibial spines and one of the surfaces
  1) lateral   2) medial

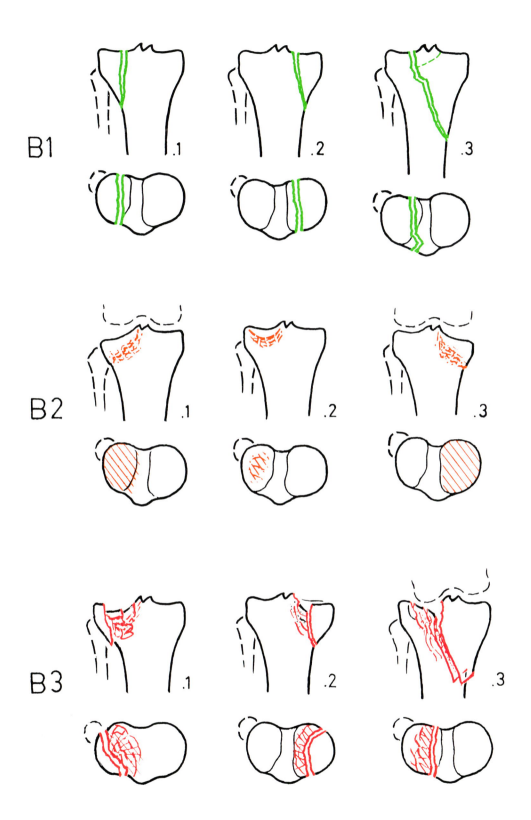

155

Subgroups of the Type C lesions can be summarized as follows:

The classification of the subgroups of the Group C1 is based on the degree of displacement of the articular fragments.

The classification of the subgroups of the Group C2, like those of the Group A3, is based on the number and the extent of the intermediate fragments. The subgroup C2.1 represents the simple articular and multifragmentary metaphyseal fractures in which the intermediate metaphyseal fragment is an intact wedge. The subgroup C2.2 represents the simple articular and multifragmentary metaphyseal fractures in which the intermediate metaphyseal fragment is a fragmented wedge. The subgroup C2.3 represents the simple articular and multifragmentary metaphyseal fractures in which the metaphyseal component is a complex fracture. C2.1 and C2.2 are further subdivided by two qualifications (1) and (2) according to whether the intermediate fragment(s) is (or are) located laterally or medially.

The subgroups of the Group C3 depend on whether the principal articular lesion is lateral, medial, or on both sides. The fractures on the lateral side have a better prognosis.

The cruciate disruption in C1 and C2 is indicated under the intercondylar eminence involvement.

Fig. 76   **C1   Complete articular fracture, articular simple, metaphyseal simple**
   1) intact anterior tibial tubercle and intercondylar eminence
   2) anterior tibial tubercle involved
   3) intercondylar eminence involved
   .1   slight displacement
   .2   one condyle displaced
   .3   both condyles displaced

C2   Complete articular fracture, articular simple, metaphyseal multifragmentary
   .1   intact wedge
      1) lateral   *2) medial*
   .2   fragmented wedge
      1) lateral   *2) medial*
   .3   complex

C3   Complete articular fracture, multifragmentary
   1) metaphyseal simple   *2) metaphyseal lateral wedge*
   3) metaphyseal medial wedge   *4) metaphyseal complex*
   5) metaphysio-diaphyseal complex
   .1   lateral
   .2   medial
   .3   lateral and medial

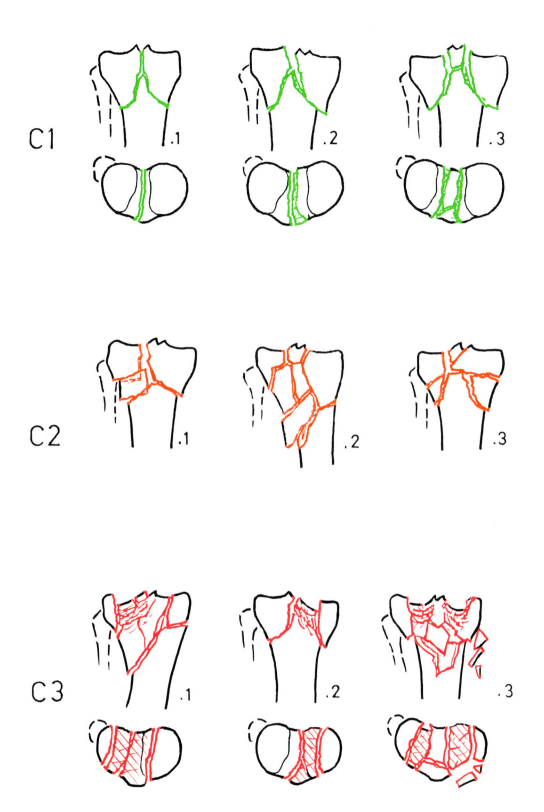

C1

    .1   .2   .3

C2

    .1   .2   .3

C3

    .1   .2   .3

4.2   Tibia/Fibula, Diaphyseal Segment = 42-

4.2.1   The Types

Fig. 77   **Tibia/Fibula diaphysis: the segment, the types**

    42-   Tibia/Fibula diaphysis
    42-A Tibia/Fibula diaphysis, simple fracture
    42-B Tibia/Fibula diaphysis, wedge fracture
    42-C Tibia/Fibula diaphysis, complex fracture

158

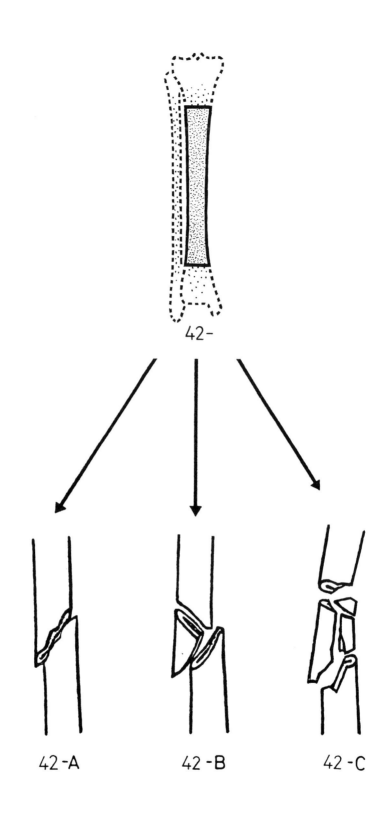

42-

42-A   42-B   42-C

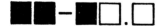

159

4.2.2   The Groups

Fig. 78   **Tibia/Fibula diaphysis: the groups**

A1   Simple fracture, spiral
A2   Simple fracture, oblique $\geq 30°$
A3   Simple fracture, transverse, $< 30°$

B1   Wedge fracture, spiral wedge
B2   Wedge fracture, bending wedge
B3   Wedge fracture, fragmented wedge

C1   Complex fracture, spiral
C2   Complex fracture, segmental
C3   Complex fracture, irregular

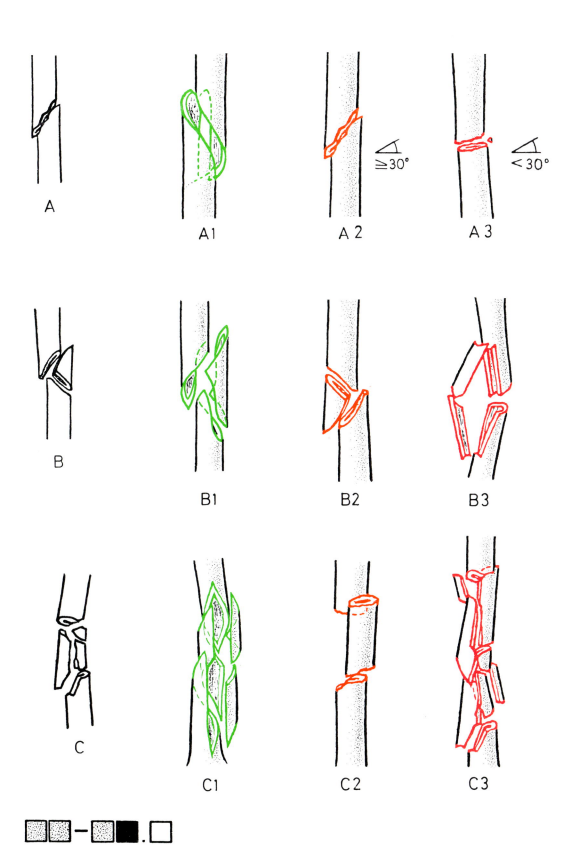

A

A1

A2 $\geqq 30°$

A3 $< 30°$

B

B1

B2

B3

C

C1

C2

C3

4.2.3   The Subgroups and Their Qualifications

Fig. 79   **Tibia/Fibula diaphysis: the subgroups and their qualifications**

A 1   Simple fracture, spiral
1) proximal zone   2) middle zone   3) distal zone
.1   fibula intact
.2   fibula fractured at another level
.3   fibula fractured at the same level

A 2   Simple fracture, oblique (≥30°)
1) proximal zone   2) middle zone   3) distal zone
.1   fibula intact
.2   fibula fractured at another level
.3   fibula fractured at the same level

A 3   Simple fracture, transverse (<30°)
1) proximal zone   2) middle zone   3) distal zone
.1   fibula intact
.2   fibula fractured at another level
.3   fibula fractured at the same level

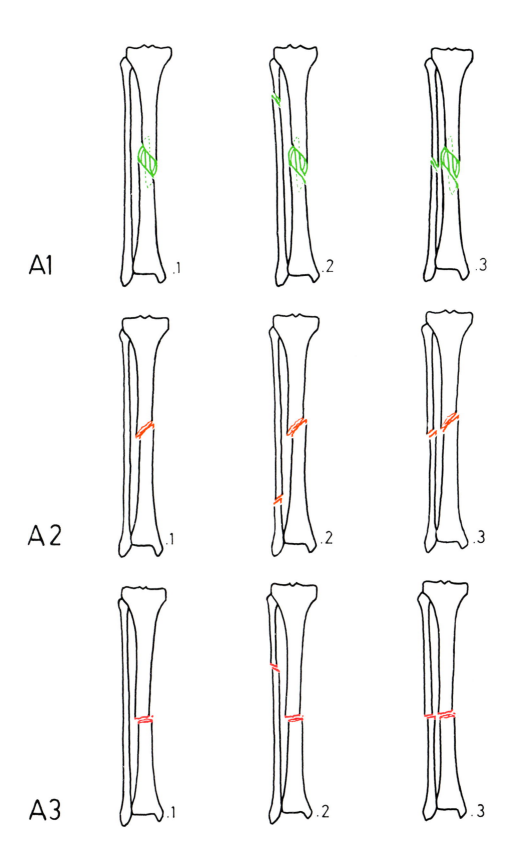

A1

.1 .2 .3

A2

.1 .2 .3

A3

.1 .2 .3

163

Fig. 80   **B1   Wedge fracture, spiral wedge**
                    1) proximal zone   2) middle zone   3) distal zone
            .1   fibula intact
            .2   fibula fractured at another level
            .3   fibula fractured at the same level

            B2   Wedge fracture, bending wedge
                    1) proximal zone   2) middle zone   3) distal zone
            .1   fibula intact
            .2   fibula fractured at another level
            .3   fibula fractured at the same level

            B3   Wedge fracture, fragmented wedge
                    1) proximal zone   2) middle zone   3) distal zone
            .1   fibula intact
            .2   fibula fractured at another level
            .3   fibula fractured at the same level

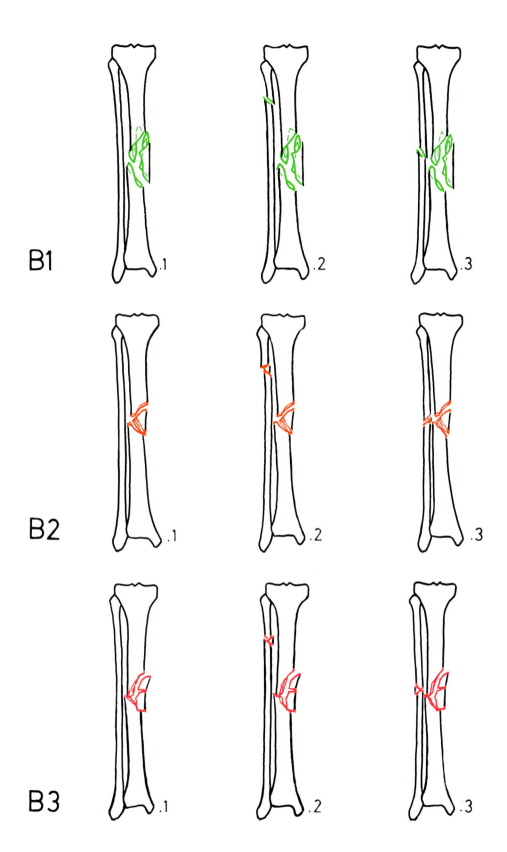

B1   .1   .2   .3

B2   .1   .2   .3

B3   .1   .2   .3

Fig. 81   **C 1**   **Complex fracture, spiral**

1) pure diaphyseal   *2) proximal diaphysio-metaphyseal*
3) distal diaphysio-metaphyseal

.1   with two intermediate fragments
.2   with three intermediate fragments
.3   with more than three intermediate fragments

C 2   **Complex fracture, segmental**

.1   with an intermediate segmental fragment

1) pure diaphyseal   *2) proximal diaphysio-metaphyseal*
3) distal diaphysio-metaphyseal   *4) oblique lines*
5) transverse and oblique lines

.2   with an intermediate segmental and additional wedge fragment(s)

1) pure diaphyseal   *2) proximal diaphysio-metaphyseal*
3) distal diaphysio-metaphyseal   *4) distal wedge*
5) three wedges, proximal and distal

.3   with two intermediate segmental fragments

1) pure diaphyseal   *2) proximal diaphysio-metaphyseal*
3) distal diaphysio-metaphyseal

C 3   **Complex fracture, irregular**

.1   with two or three intermediate fragments

1) two main intermediate fragments
2) three main intermediate fragments

.2   with limited shattering (< 4 cm)

1) proximal zone   *2) middle zone*   *3) distal zone*

.3   with extensive shattering (≥ 4 cm)

1) pure diaphyseal   *2) proximal diaphysio-metaphyseal*
3) distal diaphysio-metaphyseal

166

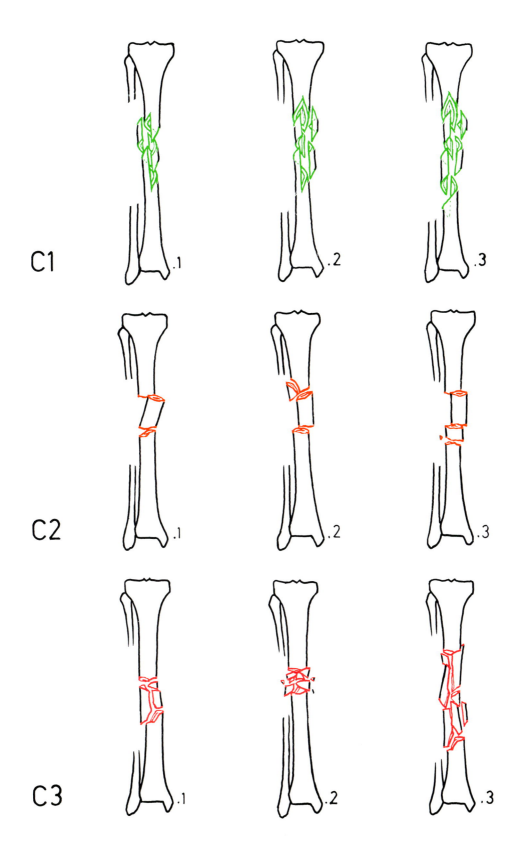

C1   .1   .2   .3

C2   .1   .2   .3

C3   .1   .2   .3

4.2.4   Comments   Evaluation of the severity scale in fractures of
                                          the tibia/fibula diaphysis.

Arrangements of the fracture groups according to their severity scale is the essence of
the AO classification of fractures. This scale was tested by our co-worker Pierre
Witschger who reviewed 400 fractures of the tibial shaft which were treated by open
reduction and internal fixation. These 400 cases were selected from an overall series
of 1000 cases. Absence of data such as the unavailability of the patient's profession
prior to fracture or failure of follow-up at one year disqualified the case for inclusion.
To ensure as much objectivity as possible, the following data were obtained from the
computer data bank at the AO Documentation Center:
1) Physician's assessment of clinical and radiologic findings on a scale from 1 to 4
(for example, 1 = no difference between the left and right leg with respect to pain, joint
function, blood supply, and axial or rotational alignment); 2) workdays missed;
3) local complications; 4) walking capacity; 5) sequence of the groups by prognosis.

Correlation of these data with the AO classification of these fractures involving the
diaphysis of the tibia, treated by open reduction and stable internal fixation and early
mobilization (fig. 82/5) showed good correspondence with the severity scale in all but
one case. The exception, the B1 fractures, ranked directly after A1, i.e. before A2 and
A3 . This was due to a lower incidence of complications. The reason for this becomes
clear if one takes into account the fact that the A1 and B1 fractures are always the
result of an indirect torsional force, whereas A2 and A3 usually result from a direct
blow. The five cases resulting in permanent disability were all type C lesions.

This study demonstrated that the scale of severity was valid in 8 out of 9 cases insofar
as surgically treated fractures of the tibia are concerned.

Fig. 82   **Evaluation of the severity scale in fractures of the tibia/fibula diaphysis
           (N = 400 cases)**

    1)   Assessment by the physician after 11-18 months (1: excellent, i.e. right = left, 2: good, 3: fair,
          4: poor)

    2)   Days of inability to work 100%

    3)   Local complications

    4)   Use of the limb less than 75% and walking ability less than 5 km

    5)   Sequence of the groups by prognosis using a summary of the tested criteria.
          Note that B-fractures are the only exception.

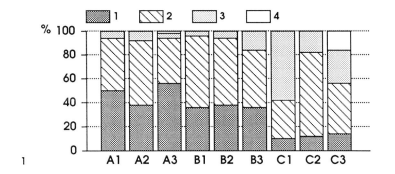

1

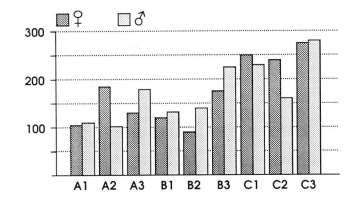

2

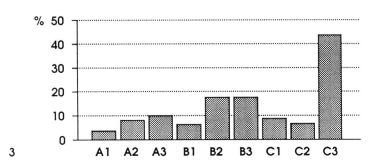

3

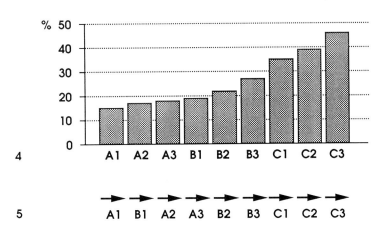

4

5   → → → → → → → → →
    A1 B1 A2 A3 B2 B3 C1 C2 C3

4.3 Tibia/Fibula, Distal Segment = 43-

4.3.1 The Types

This segment is defined by the square method. We distinguish three fracture types in this segment. These are: **Type A**, the extra-articular fractures, **Type B**, the partial articular fractures which involve only part of the distal articular surface of the tibia, and **Type C**, the complete articular fractures in which the distal articular surface is divided into at least two fragments which are completely detached from the diaphysis.

Type B and C lesions fit under the heading of "fractures of the tibial plafond" or "pilon fractures".

Fig. 83   **Tibia/Fibula distal: the bone, the segment, and the types**

4   Tibia/Fibula
43-   Tibia/Fibula distal
43-A   Tibia/Fibula distal, extra-articular fracture
43-B   Tibia/Fibula distal, partial articular fracture
43-C   Tibia/Fibula distal, complete articular fracture

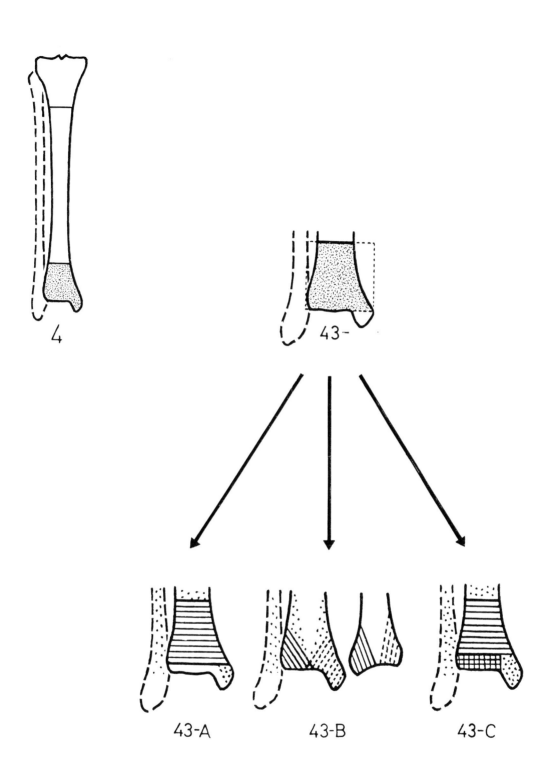

4

43-

43-A   43-B   43-C

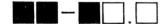

171

4.3.2 The Groups

The Type A fractures, i.e. the extra-articular fractures, can be divided into three groups in an ascending order of severity depending on the shape of the metaphyseal fracture and the number and the extent of the intermediate fragments. **A1** are the simple fractures, **A2** the metaphyseal wedge fractures, and **A3** the metaphyseal complex fractures.

The Type B fractures, i.e. the partial articular fractures, are classified according to the shape and the extent of the articular surface involvement. **B1** represent a simple disruption of the articular surface. These are the "pure split fractures". In **B2** the articular surface exhibits not only a simple fracture line but also a depressed area of the articular surface in which the fragments remain contiguous like in a mosaic; these are the "split-depression fractures". In **B3** the articular surface is broken into several fragments; these are referred to as "multifragmentary depression fractures".

The Type C fractures, i.e. the complete articular fractures, are classified according to the degree of articular and metaphyseal involvement. In **C1**, i.e. the simple articular and simple metaphyseal fractures, both the articular surface and the metaphysis display simple fracture lines. In **C2**, i.e. the simple articular and multifragmentary metaphyseal fractures, the articular surface displays a simple fracture line but there is impaction at the level of the metaphysis. In **C3**, the complete articular multifragmentary fractures, the articular surface and, in most cases, the metaphysis display multiple fractures.

Fig. 84   **Tibia/Fibula distal: the groups**

A1   Extra-articular fracture, metaphyseal simple
A2   Extra-articular fracture, metaphyseal wedge
A3   Extra-articular fracture, metaphyseal complex

B1   Partial articular fracture, pure split
B2   Partial articular fracture, split-depression
B3   Partial articular fracture, multifragmentary depression

C1   Complete articular fracture, articular simple, metaphyseal simple
C2   Complete articular fracture, articular simple, metaphyseal multifragmentary
C3   Complete articular fracture, multifragmentary

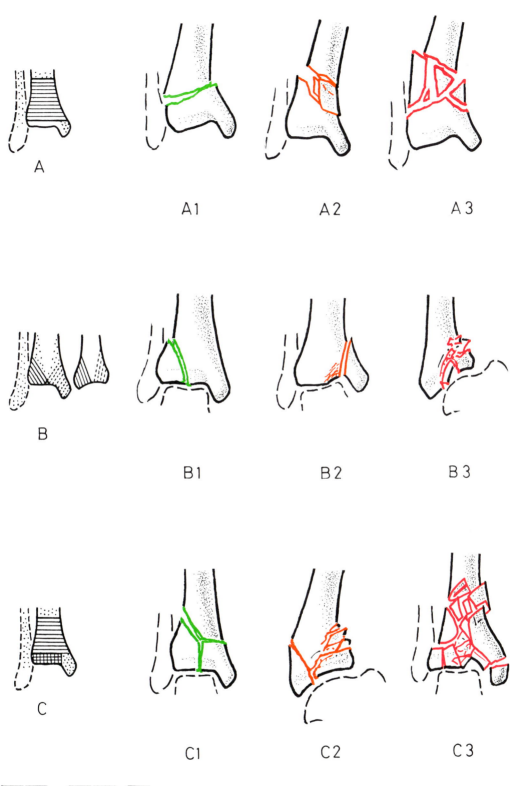

A

A1 A2 A3

B

B1 B2 B3

C

C1 C2 C3

173

4.3.3 The Subgroups and Their Qualifications

Please note: All the qualifications of the subgroups of the distal tibia are identical. They all describe the associated lesions of the fibula.

Fig. 85 **Tibia/Fibula distal: the subgroups and their qualifications**

A 1 Extra-articular fracture, metaphyseal simple
          1) fibula intact   2) simple fracture of the fibula
          3) multifragmentary fracture of the fibula
          4) bifocal fracture of the fibula
  .1   spiral
  .2   oblique
  .3   transverse

A 2 Extra-articular fracture, metaphyseal wedge
          1) fibula intact   2) simple fracture of the fibula
          3) multifragmentary fracture of the fibula
          4) bifocal fracture of the fibula
  .1   postero-lateral impaction
  .2   antero-medial wedge
  .3   extending into the diaphysis

A 3 Extra-articular fracture, metaphyseal complex
          1) fibula intact   2) simple fracture of the fibula
          3) multifragmentary fracture of the fibula
          4) bifocal fracture of the fibula
  .1   three intermediate fragments
  .2   more than three intermediate fragments
  .3   extending into the diaphysis

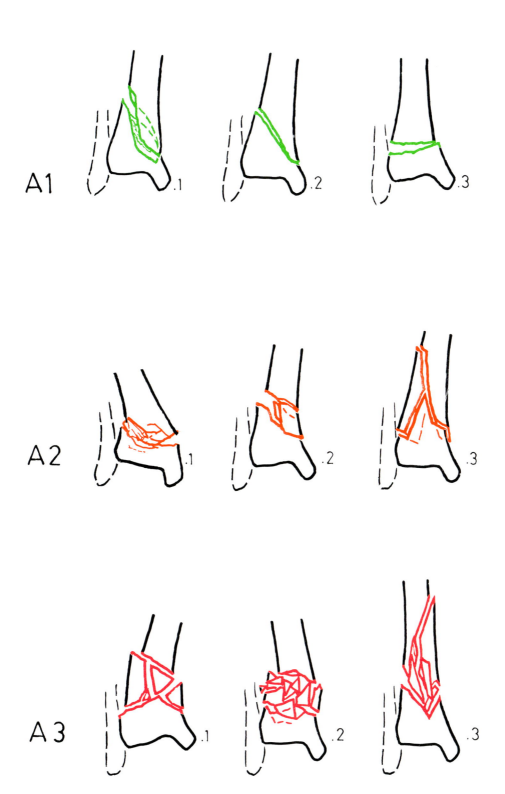

A1

.1   .2   .3

A2

.1   .2   .3

A3

.1   .2   .3

175

Please note: Split-depression of the central fragment = B2.3:
Depression of the entire fragment between or within the two splits.

Fig. 86   **B1   Partial articular fracture, pure split**
 1) fibula intact   *2) simple fracture of the fibula*
 3) multifragmentary fracture of the fibula
 4) bifocal fracture of the fibula

 .1   frontal   *5) anterior*   *6) posterior (Volkmann)*
 .2   sagittal   *5) lateral*   *6) medial (medial malleolus)*
 .3   metaphyseal multifragmentary

B2   Partial articular fracture, split-depression
 1) fibula intact   *2) simple fracture of the fibula*
 3) multifragmentary fracture of the fibula
 4) bifocal fracture of the fibula

 .1   frontal   *5) anterior*   *6) posterior*
 .2   sagittal   *5) lateral*   *6) medial*
 .3   of the central fragment

B3   Partial articular fracture, multifragmentary depression
 1) fibula intact   *2) simple fracture of the fibula*
 3) multifragmentary fracture of the fibula
 4) bifocal fracture of the fibula

 .1   frontal   *5) anterior*   *6) posterior*
 .2   sagittal   *5) lateral*   *6) medial*
 .3   metaphyseal multifragmentary

B1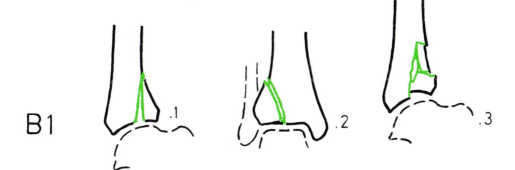

B2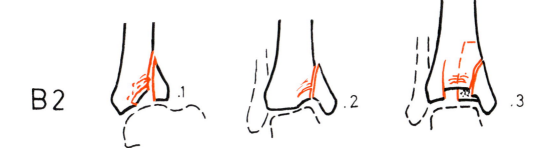

B3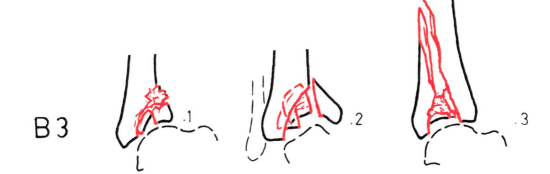

Please note: Small depressions of the articulation (10-20%) are common to the fractures C1.2 and .3, C2.2 and .3.

Fig. 87   **C 1   Complete articular fracture, articular simple, metaphyseal simple**
1) fibula intact   2) simple fracture of the fibula
3) multifragmentary fracture of the fibula
4) bifocal fracture of the fibula
.1   without impaction   *5) frontal plane   6) sagittal plane*
.2   with epiphyseal depression
.3   extending into the diaphysis

C 2   Complete articular fracture, articular simple, metaphyseal multifragmentary
1) fibula intact   2) simple fracture of the fibula
3) multifragmentary fracture of the fibula
4) bifocal fracture of the fibula
.1   with asymmetric impaction   *5) frontal plane split   6) sagittal plane split*
.2   without asymmetric impaction
.3   extending into the diaphysis

C 3   Complete articular fracture, multifragmentary
1) fibula intact   2) simple fracture of the fibula
3) multifragmentary fracture of the fibula
4) bifocal fracture of the fibula
.1   epiphyseal
.2   epiphysio-metaphyseal
.3   epiphysio-metaphysio-diaphyseal

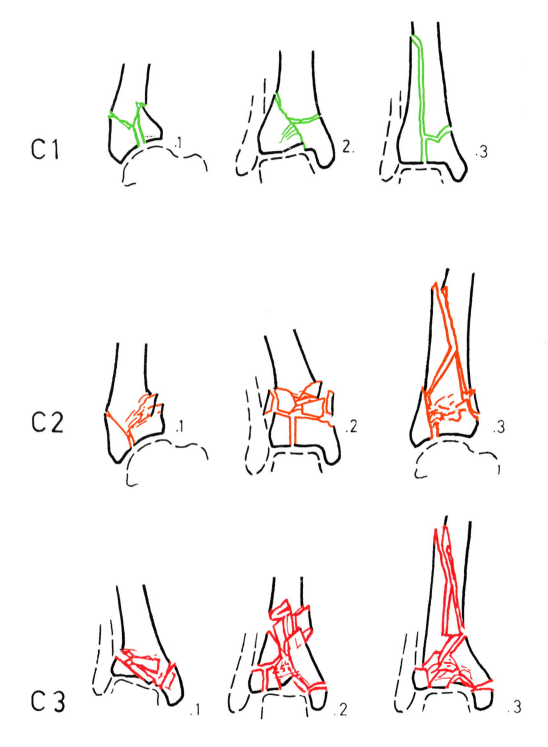

C 1   .1   .2   .3

C 2   .1   .2   .3

C 3   .1   .2   .3

179

4.4   Tibia/Fibula, Malleolar Segment = 44-

4.4.1   The Types

The malleolar fractures are considered as a separate segment: 44-. Like fractures of
the other segments, they are divided into three lesion types: A, B, and C . This divi-
sion is based on the level of the lateral malleolar lesion in relation to the level of the
syndesmotic ligament complex.

In the **Type A**, the lateral lesion is below the syndesmotic ligament ; these lesions are
referred to as "infrasyndesmotic". In the **Type B**, the fracture of the fibula is between
the anterior and posterior tibio-fibular or syndesmotic ligaments. These fractures are
refered to as "trans-syndesmotic". In the **Type C** the lateral lesion is above the
syndesmotic ligaments. These lesions are referred to as "supra-syndesmotic".

> **Please note:**
> - The fractures of the posterior articular margins (Volkmann) without lesion of the fibula are
> considered as fractures of the distal tibia: 43-B1.1 (6)
> - The fractures of the medial malleolus without lesions of the fibula are classified in the distal
> tibia fractures: 43-B1.2 (6)

Fig. 88   **Tibia/Fibula, Malleolar Segment: the bone, and the types**

4   Tibia/Fibula
44-   Tibia/Fibula, malleolar segment
44-A   Tibia/Fibula, malleolar segment, infrasydesmotic lesion
44-B   Tibia/Fibula, malleolar segment, transsyndesmotic fibula fracture
44-C   Tibia/Fibula, malleolar segment, suprasyndesmotic lesion

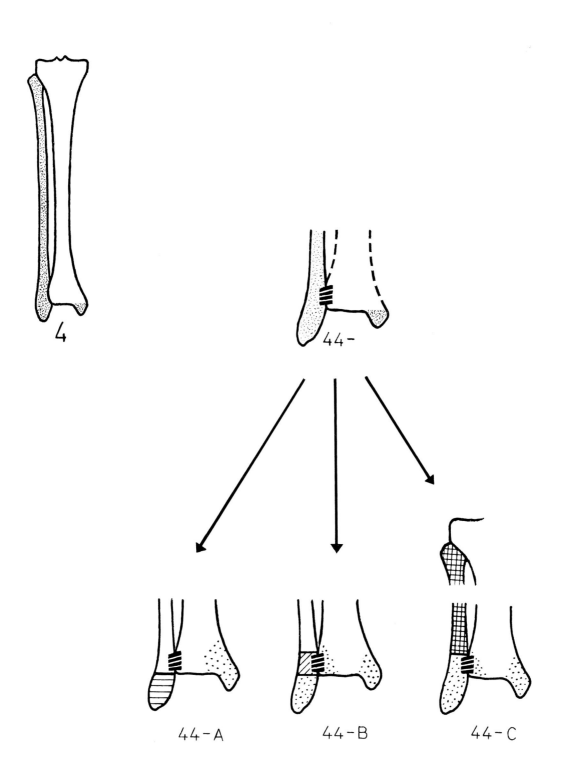

44-A   44-B   44-C

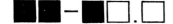

4.4.2   The Groups

The Type A lesions are classified into three **groups** which are: **A1** if the lateral infra-syndesmotic lesion is isolated, **A2** if the lateral infra-syndesmotic lesion is associated with a fracture of the medial malleolus, and as **A3** if the lateral infrasyndesmotic lesion is associated with a fracture of the medial malleolus with a postero-medial extension.

The Type B lesions are classified into three **groups** which are: **B1** if the transsyndesmotic fibular fracture is isolated, **B2** if the transsyndesmotic fracture of the fibula is associated with a fracture on the medial malleolus, and **B3** if the trans-syndesmotic fracture of the fibula is associated with a fracture of the medial malleolus with a complete rupture of the syndesmotic ligament.

The Type C fractures all have a fracture of the fibula which is above the syndesmosis. They are classified therefore on the basis of the **type** and the **level** of the fibular lesion. The three groups are as follows: **C1** if the fibular shaft displays a simple fracture, **C2** if the fibular diaphysis fracture is multifragmentary, and **C3** if the fibular shaft lesion is located at the proximal end of the fibula (neck or head fracture or proximal tibio-fibular dislocation).

Please note:
Total rupture of the syndesmosis corresponds to a rupture of the anterior and posterior tibio-fibular ligaments. This can result either from a rupture of the ligaments themselves or from an avulsion of the attachment of the ligament from bone. The detachment of the medial insertion of the anterior syndesmotic ligament from the anterior tibial tuberosity is known as the "Tillaux-Chaput" lesion (or simply "**Chaput**") and the detachment or avulsion of the posterior margin or tuberosity is known as the "Volkmann fracture" (or simply "**Volkmann**"). The detachment of the anterior insertion of the anterior syndesmotic ligament from the lateral malleollus, if it occurs with an avulsion, is known as the "Le Fort fracture" (or simply "**Le Fort**").
The **rupture of the anterior syndesmosis** can be either a disruption of the anterior tibio-fibular ligament or an avulsion of the attachment of the anterior tibio-fibular ligament, either from the tibia ("Chaput") or from the lateral malleolus ("Le Fort").

Fig. 89   **Tibia/Fibula, Malleolar Segment: the groups**

A1   Infrasyndesmotic lesion, isolated
A2   Infrasyndesmotic lesion, with a fracture of the medial malleolus
A3   Infrasyndesmotic lesion, with a postero-medial fracture

B1   Transsyndesmotic fibula fracture, isolated
B2   Transsyndesmotic fibula fracture, with a medial lesion
B3   Transsyndesmotic fibula fracture, with a medial lesion and Volkmann (fracture of the postero-lateral rim)

C1   Suprasyndesmotic lesion, diaphyseal fracture of the fibula, simple
C2   Suprasyndesmotic lesion, diaphyseal fracture of the fibula, multifragmentary
C3   Suprasyndesmotic lesion, proximal fibula

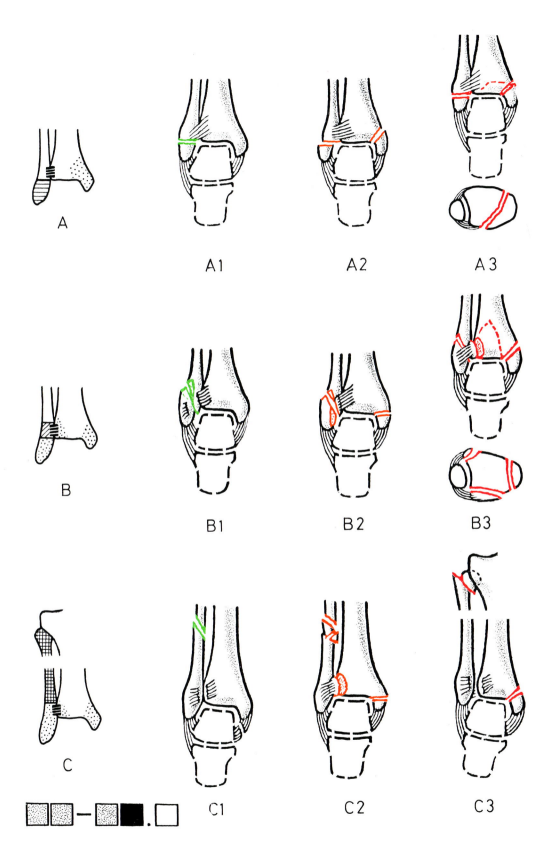

A

A1   A2   A3

B

B1   B2   B3

C

C1   C2   C3

183

4.4.3   The Subgroups and Their Qualifications

The Group **A1** are all the unifocal lateral lesions, i.e. all the isolated lesions of the lateral malleollus or of the lateral collateral ligament. The Group **A2** includes all the bifocal lesions, i.e. the fractures of the lateral and medial malleollus. The Group **A3** includes the circumferential lesions, i.e. the fractures of the lateral and medial malleolus in which the fracture of the medial malleolus always has a posterior marginal extension.

The lateral lesion in all the Type A fractures is the same in the corresponding sub-groups. Thus the **subgroup** .1 is a rupture of the lateral collateral ligament, .2 is an avulsion of the tip of the lateral malleolus, and the subgroup .3 is a transverse fracture of the lateral malleolus below the syndesmotic ligament.
In A2 the three qualifications describe the direction of the fracture of the medial malleolus.

Fig. 90   **Tibia/Fibula, Malleolar Segment: the subgroups and their qualifications**

A1   Infrasyndesmotic lesion, isolated
  .1   rupture of the lateral collateral ligament
  .2   avulsion of the tip of the lateral malleolus
  .3   transverse fracture of the lateral malleolus

A2   Infrasyndesmotic lesion, with fracture of the medial malleolus
          1) transverse   2) oblique   3) vertical
  .1   rupture of the lateral collateral ligament
  .2   avulsion of the tip of the lateral malleolus
  .3   transverse fracture of the lateral malleolus

A3   Infrasyndesmotic lesion, with postero-medial fracture
  .1   rupture of the lateral collateral ligament
  .2   avulsion of the tip of the lateral malleolus
  .3   transverse fracture of the lateral malleolus

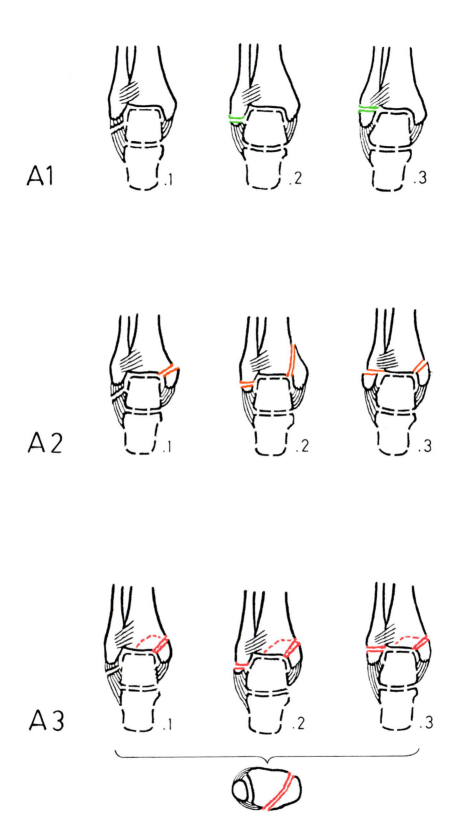

A1   .1   .2   .3

A2   .1   .2   .3

A3   .1   .2   .3

185

Type **B** lesions, i.e. transsyndesmotic fibular fractures, are classified as B1 if the lesion involves only the lateral side of the joint, as B2 if it involves the lateral and the medial sides, and as B3 if it involves the lateral, the medial and the posterior sides.

All these lesions may have an associated rupture of the anterior syndesmotic ligament, at least partially. This is denoted by the appropriate qualification, as an in-substance rupture or an avulsion from the tibia (Chaput), or as an avulsion from the lateral malleolus (Le Fort).

The three qualifications of B3 relate to the Volkmann lesion.

Fig. 91   **B1**   **Transsyndesmotic fibular fracture, isolated**
        .1   simple
        .2   simple, with rupture of the anterior syndesmosis
                1) in-substance   *2) Chaput*   *3) Le Fort*
        .3   multifragmentary

    B2   **Transsyndesmotic fibular fracture, with medial lesion**
        .1   simple, with rupture of the medial collateral ligament and rupture of the anterior syndesmosis
                1) in substance   *2) Chaput*   *3) Le Fort*
        .2   simple, with fracture of the medial malleolus and with rupture of the anterior syndesmosis
                1) in-substance   *2) Chaput*   *3) Le Fort*
        .3   multifragmentary
                1) and rupture of the medial collateral ligament
                2) and fracture of the medial malleolus

    B3   **Transsyndesmotic fibular fracture, with medial lesion and a Volkmann (fracture of the postero-lateral rim)**
                1) extra-articular avulsion   *2) peripheral articular fragment*
                3) significant articular fragment
        .1   fibula simple, with rupture of the medial collateral ligament
        .2   fibula simple, with fracture of the medial malleolus
        .3   fibula multifragmentary, with fracture of the medial malleolus

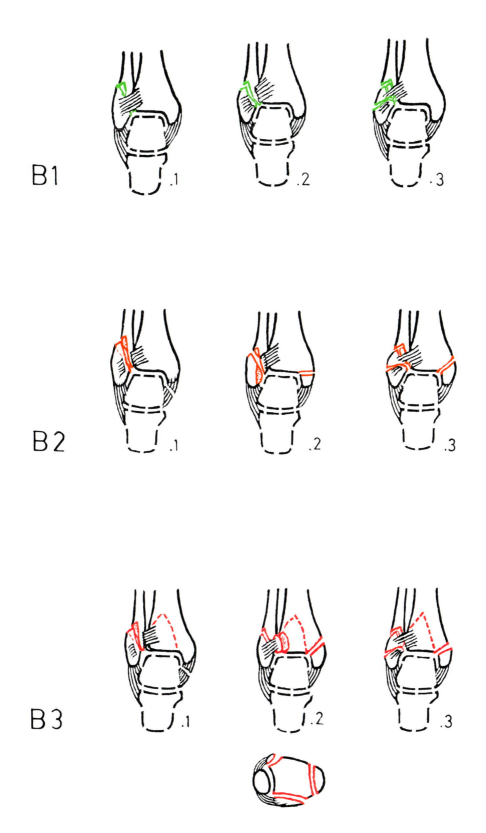

B1

  .1   .2   .3

B2

  .1   .2   .3

B3

  .1   .2   .3

? not always according to nich Gjelli

Type C fractures always have a bifocal lesion and the syndesmosis is always disrupted at least anteriorly. If a Volkmann lesion is involved, the fracture of the posterior tibial margin (posterior tuberosity) may or not be articular. A Volkmann lesion is always present in the **subgroup** .3 as C1.3, C2.3, and C3.3. The qualification is used to indicate whether the Volkmann lesion is *(1) an extra-articular avulsion, (2) an articular rim fragment or (3) a large articular fragment.*

The fracture of the fibular diaphysis is simple in C1 and multifragmentary in C2. In C3 this lateral lesion is proximal *[fracture through the neck (1) or through the head (2), or tibio-fibular dislocation].* When all the attachments between the tibia and fibula are broken, the head of the fibula is always pushed up and a dislocation of the proximal tibio-fibular joint is the rule (see C3.3(3)).

Fig. 92   **C 1   Suprasyndesmotic lesion, diaphyseal fracture of the fibula, simple**
     .1   with rupture of the medial collateral ligament
     .2   with fracture of the medial malleolus
     .3   with fracture of the medial malleolus and a Volkmann (= Dupuytren)
           1) extra-articular avulsion   2) peripheral articular fragment
           3) significant articular fragment

C 2   Suprasyndesmotic lesion, diaphyseal fracture of the fibula, multifragmentary
     .1   with rupture of the medial collateral ligament
     .2   with fracture of the medial malleolus
     .3   with fracture of the medial malleolus and a Volkmann (= Dupuytren)
           1) extra-articular avulsion   2) peripheral articular fragment
           3) significant articular fragment

C 3   Suprasyndesmotic lesion, proximal fibular lesion
           1) fracture through the neck
           2) fracture through the head
           3) proximal tibio-fibular dislocation
           4) rupture of the medial collateral ligament
           5) fracture of the medial malleolus
           6) articular fragment
     .1   without shortening, without Volkmann
     .2   with shortening, without Volkmann
     .3   medial lesion and a Volkmann

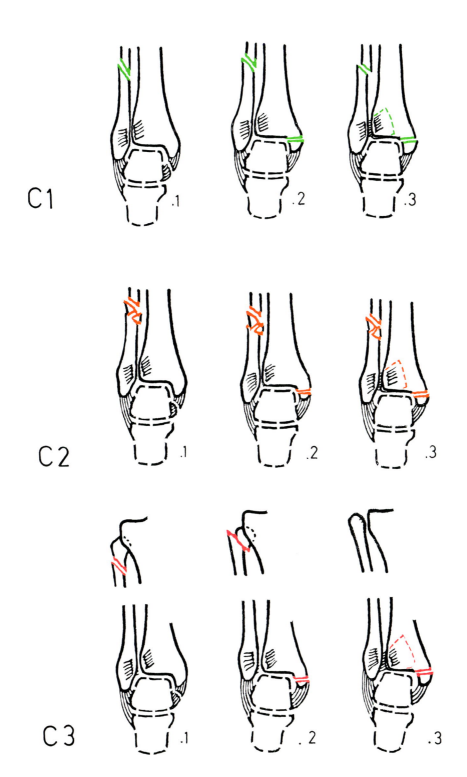

C1   .1   .2   .3

C2   .1   .2   .3

C3   .1   .2   .3

4.4.4   Comments about Malleolar Fractures

Four structures are essential for the classification of fractures involving the malleoli. These are:

1) The **fibula**. The level of the fibular lesion determines the fracture type. Type A fractures are located below the syndesmosis, Type B are located at the level of the syndesmosis, and Type C are located above the syndesmosis.

2) The **anterior syndesmosis** or **anterior tibio-fibular ligament**. The ligament itself may be disrupted in its substance or it may be avulsed with the anterior tibial tuberosity ("Tillaux-Chaput" lesion or simply "**Chaput**") or from the lateral malleolus ("Le Fort" lesion or simply "**Le Fort**").

3) The **medial malleolus**. The medial lesion can be a disruption of the ligament, an avulsion of the malleolar tip, or a transverse, an oblique or a vertical fracture of the medial malleolus. This pattern depends on the mechanism of the fracture.

4) The **posterior syndesmosis** or the **posterior tibio-fibular ligament**. The in-substance disruption of the posterior tibio-fibular ligament is a fairly infrequent injury. The avulsion of the posterior tuberosity ("Volkmann lesion" or simply "**Volkmann**") can be only a cortical avulsion but more commonly it is a larger fragment containing a variable amount of the posterior articular rim (for isolated Volkmann see also notes page 180).

Fig. 93   **The four essential structures for the classification of the lesions of the malleolar segment**

1)   **The lateral lesion determines the fracture type** (marked zones)
   A)   infrasyndesmotic = below the syndesmosis
   B)   transsyndesmotic = at the level of the syndesmosis
   C)   suprasyndesmotic = above the syndesmosis

2)   **Anterior syndesmosis = anterior tibio-fibular ligament**
   a)   rupture of the substance of the ligament
   b)   avulsion from the tibia = "Chaput" lesion
   c)   avulsion from the lateral malleolus = "Le Fort" lesion

3)   **Fracture of the medial malleolus**
   a)   avulsion of the tip
   b)   transverse
   c)   oblique
   d)   vertical

4)   **Fracture of the posterior tuberosity = "Volkmann" lesion**
   a)   extra-articular, cortical avulsion
   b)   intra-articular, small fragment
   c)   intra-articular, large fragment

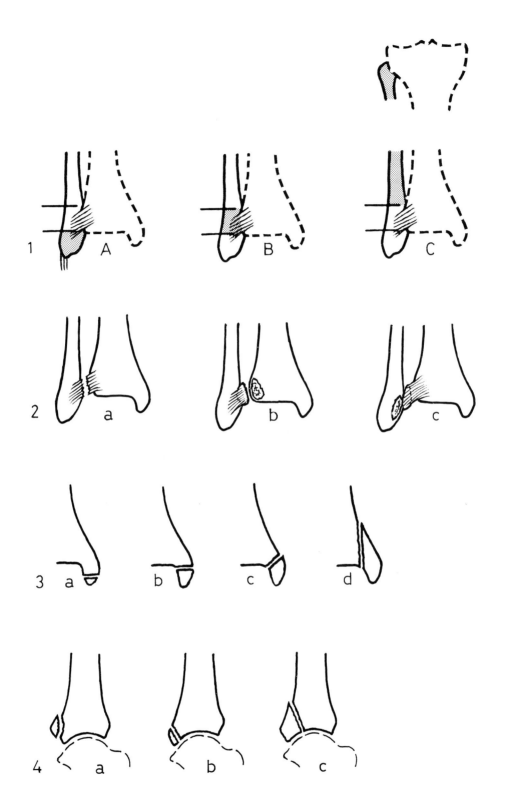

191

Bibliography Concerning the Long Bones

(works and articles that have been studied, classified according to the segment)

Generalities:

Böhler, L.: Technique du traitement des fractures. Paris: Éditions Médicales France 1944.

Heim, U.F.A., Pfeiffer, K.M.: Ostéosynthèses périphériques à l'aide de l'instrumentation pour petits fragments de l'AO. Paris: Masson 1975.

Heim, U.F.A., Pfeiffer, K.M.: Internal fixation of small fractures. Techniques recommended by the AO-ASIF group. 3rd ed. Berlin-Heidelberg-New York: Springer-Verlag 1988.

Heim, U.F.A.: Die Grenzziehung zwischen Diaphyse und Metaphyse mit Hilfe der Viereckmessung. Ein Beitrag zur Klassifizierung und Dokumentierung von Frakturen der langen Röhrenknochen am Beispiel der distalen Tibia. *Unfallchirurg 90:274-280 (1987)*

Müller, M.E.: Klassifikation und internationale AO-Dokumentation der Femurfrakturen. *Unfallheilkunde 83:251 (1980).*

Müller, M.E., Allgöwer, M., Schneider, R., Willenegger, H.: Manual der Osteosynthese. AO-Technik, 2. Aufl. Berlin-Heidelberg-New York: Springer-Verlag 1977.

Müller, M.E., Allgöwer, M., Schneider, R., Willenegger, H.: Manual of Internal Fixation. Techniques recommended by the AO-Group. Second Edition. Berlin-Heidelberg-New York: Springer-Verlag 1979.

Müller, M.E., Koch, P., Zehnder, R.: Computerized Documentation of Fractures. Scientific Exhibits, 52nd Annual Meeting A.A.O.S., Las Vegas, January 1985.

Müller, M.E.: Letter to the Editor of the S.I.C.O.T. Newsletter. *Int Orthop Newsletter N°7 (1988)*

Rockwood, C.A., Green, D.P. (Editors): Fractures. Philadelphia-Toronto: Lippincott 1975.

11- Dubousset, J.: Luxations postérieures de l'épaule. *Rev. Chir. orthop. 53:65 (1967).*

Duparc, J., Largier, A.: Les luxations-fractures de l'extrémité supérieure de l'humérus. *Rev Chir orthop 62:91 (1976).*

Jakob, R.P., Kristiansen, T., Mayo, K., Ganz, R., and Müller, M.E.: Classification and aspects of treatment of fractures of the proximal humerus. In: Surgery of the Shoulder (Bateman, J.E. and Welsh, R.P., ed.), p. 330. Philadelphia-Toronto: Decker 1984.

Neer, Ch.S.: Displaced proximal humerus fractures. *J Bone Jt Surg 52-A:1077 (1970).*

Neer, Ch.S.: Fractures about the Shoulder. In: Fractures in Adults (Rockwood, Ch.A., Green, D.P., ed.al.), p. 675. Philadelphia: Lippincott Company 1984.

Neer, Ch.S., Brown, T.H., McLaughlin, H.L.: Fracture of the neck of the humerus with dislocation of the head fragment. *Am J Surgery, p. 252 (1953).*

Olivier, H.: Fractures de l'extrémité supérieure de l'humérus. *Encycl Médico-Chirurgicale (Paris) 14038 A[10].*

Oliver, H., Dufour, G., Duparc, J.: Les fractures du trochiter. *Rev Chir orthop 62, Suppl.113 (1976).*

Razemon, J.-P., Baux, S.: Les fractures et les fractures-luxations de l'extrémité supérieure de l'humérus. *Rev Chir orthop 55:388 (1969).*

13- Benoit, J., Dupont, J.Y., Lecestre ed al.: Techniques opératoires du coude. *Encycl Médico-Chirurgicale (Paris) 44325.*

Castaing, J., et le club des dix: Les fractures récentes de l'extrémité inférieure du radius chez l'adulte. *Rev Chir orthop 50:581 (1964).*

Hahn, N.F.: Fall von einer Varietät der Frakturen des Ellbogens. *Z. Wundärzte und Geburtshilfe 6:185 (1853).*

Judet, R.: Le traitement des fractures de l'extrémité inférieure de l'humérus chez l'adulte. *Rev Chir orthop 50, 3:275 (1964).*

Kocher, T.: Beiträge zur Kenntnis einiger praktisch wichtiger Fracturformen. Basel-Leipzig: Sallmann 1896.

Lance, D., Seringe, R.: Les fractures de l'extrémité inférieure de l'humérus de l'enfant. *Encycl Médico-Chirurgicale (Paris)* ***14041 B***[10].

Lecestre, P.: Les fractures de l'extrémité inférieure de l'humérus chez l'adulte. SO.F.C.O.T. Réunion annuelle, nov. 1979, *Rev Chir orthop 66, Suppl. II:21 (1980).*

Lecestre, P., Dupont, J.Y., Lortat, J.A., Ramadier, J.O.: Les fractures complexes de l'extrémité inférieure de l'humérus chez l'adulte. A propos de 66 cas dont 55 opérés. *Rev Chir orthop **65**:11 (1979).*

Marion, J., Faysse, R., Lagrange, J., Rigault, P.: Les fractures de l'extrémité inférieure de l'humérus chez l'enfant. *Rev Chir orthop **48**:333 (1962).*

Mestdagh, H., Sensey, J.J., Fontaine, C., Giard, H.: Luxations du coude. *Encycl Médico-Chirurgicale (Paris) 14042 A*[10].

Milch, H.: Fractures and Fracture Dislocations of the Humeral Condyles. *J Trauma 4:592(1964).*

Pidhorz, L., Beddouk, A.: Fractures de la palette humérale de l'adulte. *Encycl Médico-Chirurgicale (Paris)* ***14041 A***[10].

Riseborough, E.Y., Radin, E.L.: Intercondylar T-fractures of the Humerus in the Adult. (A Comparison of Operative and Non-operative Treatment in Twentynine Cases).*J Bone Jt Surg **51-A**:130 (1969).*

21- Allieu, Y., Vidal, J.: Fractures de l'extrémité supérieure des deux os de l'avant-bras. *Encycl Médico-Chirurgicale (Paris)* ***14042 B***[10].

Radin, E.L., Riseborough, E.J.: Fractures of the Radial Head. A Review of Eighty-eight Cases and Analysis of the Indications for Excision of the Radial Head and Non-Operative Treatment. *J Bone Jt Surg **48-A**:1055 (1966).*

22- Boucher, R., Witvoét, J.: Fractures diaphysaires de l'avant-bras. *Encycl Médico-Chirurgicale (Paris)* ***14044 B***[10].

Gross, E.: Osteosynthese bei Vorderarmschaftfrakturen. *AO-Bulletin 1979.*

Mikic, Z.D.: Galeazzi Fracture-Dislocations. *J. Bone Jt Surg. **57-A**:1071 (1975).*

Raux, P., Finidori, G., Lesaux, D., et al.: Fracture de Monteggia chez l'enfant (Étude de 57 cas). *Ann Chir Infantile **16**:423 (1975).*

Trillat, A., Marsan, C., Lapeyre, B.: Classification et traitement des fractures de Monteggia. A propos de 36 observations. *Rev Chir orthop **55**:639 (1969).*

23- Duparc, J., Valtin, B.: Fractures de l'extrémité inférieure des deux os de l'avant-bras de l'adulte. *Encycl Médico-Chirurgicale (Paris)* ***14045 B***[10].

Fernandez, D.L.: Correction of post-traumatic wrist deformity in adults by osteotomy, bone-grafting, and internal fixation. *J Bone Jt. Surg **64-A**:1164 (1982).*

31- Barnes, R., Brown, J.T., Garden, R.S., Nicoll, E.A.: Subcapital fractures of the femur. A prospective review. *J Bone Jt Surg. **58-B**:2 (1976).*

Decoulx, P., Lavarde, G.: Les fractures de la région trochantérienne. Étude statistique sur 2´612 observations. *J. Chir (Paris) **98**:75 (1969).*

Garden, R.S.: Stability and union in subcapital fractures of the femur. *J Bone Jt Surg **46-B**:630 (1964).*

Garden, R.S.: Malreduction and avascular necrosis in subcapital fractures of the femur. *J Bone Jt Surg **53-B**:183 (1971).*

Jeanmaire, E.: La fracture du col du fémur. Étude analytique par un nouveau procédé informatique. Thèse pour l'obtention du Doctorat de la Faculté de Médecine de l'Université de Berne, mai 1981.

Kempf, I.: Fractures de l'extrémité supérieure du fémur. Cahiers d'enseignement de la SO.F.C.O.T.. Paris: Expansion scientifique française 1980.

Letenneur, J., Rogez, J.M., Leveau, J., Maulaz, D.: Luxations traumatiques pures de la hanche. Luxations de hanche et fractures de tête fémorale. *Encycl Médico-Chirurgicale (Paris) 14077 A*[10].

Lord, G., Samuel, P.: Fractures de l'extrémité supérieure du fémur. *Encycl Médico-Chirurgicale (Paris)* **14076 A**[10].

Pipkin, G.: Treatment of Grade IV Fracture-Dislocation of the Hip. A Review. *J Bone Jt Surg* **39-A:1027 (1957)**.

Ricard, R., Molé, L.: Les fractures cervicales vraies récentes du fémur. SO.F.C.O.T. Réunion annuelle, nov. 1965. *Rev Chir orthop* **51:326 (1965)**.

Rigault, P., Iselin, F., Moreau, J., Judet, J.: Fractures du col du fémur chez l'enfant (Étude de 25 cas). *Rev Chir orthop* **52:325 (1966)**.

Weigand, H., Schweikert, C.-H., Strube, H.-D.: Die traumatische Hüftluxation mit Hüftkopfkalottenfraktur. *Unfallheilkunde* **81:377 (1978)**.

32- Pidhorz, L., Moreau, P.: Fractures de la diaphyse fémorale de l'adulte. *Encycl Médico-Chirurgicale (Paris)* **14078 A**[10].

33- Blaimont, P., Simons, M.: Le traitement des fractures basses du fémur chez l'adulte. Rapport Congrès annuel Soc.Belge d'Orthopédie, de Traumatologie et de Chir. App. Moteur, mai 1970. *Acta Orthop Belg* **36:1 (1970)**.

Gérard, Y.: Fractures de l'extrémité inférieure du fémur. *Encycl Médico-Chirurgicale (Paris)* **14080 A**[10].

Moore, T.M.: Fracture-Dislocation of the Knee. *Clin. Orthop. related Res.* **156:128 (1981)**.

Neer, Ch.S., Grantham, S.A., Shelton, M.L.: Supracondylar Fracture of the Adult Femur. *J Bone Jt Surg* **49-A, 4:591 (1967)**.

Seinsheimer, F.: Fractures of the Distal Femur. *Clin Orthop* **153:169 (1980)**.

Trillat, A., Dejour, H., Bost, J., Nourissat, Ch.: Les fractures unicondyliennes du fémur. *Rev Chir orthop* **61:611 (1975)**.

41- Bousquet, G., Rhenter, J.L., Bascoulergue, G., Millon, J.: Fractures des épines tibiales. *Encycl Médico-Chirurgicale (Paris)* **14082 B**[10].

Duparc, J., Ficat, P.: Fractures articulaires de l'extrémité supérieure du tibia. *Rev chir orthop* **46:399 (1960)**.

Hohl, M.: Tibial Condylar Fractures. *J Bone Jt Surg* **49-A, 1455 (1967)**.

Schatzker, J., McBroom, R., Bruce, D.: The Tibial Plateau Fracture. *Clin Orthop* **138:94, 1979**.

42- Cauchoix, J., Duparc, J., Deburge, A., Caracostas, M.: Sur le traitement primitif et secondaire des fractures fermées de jambe. *Rev Chir orthop* **51:469 (1965)**.

Johner, R.: Die Unterschenkelschaftfraktur. Unfallmechanismus, Morphologie und Klassifikation. *Helv Chir Acta* **49:237 (1982)**.

Johner, R., Wruhs, O.: Classification of Tibial Shaft Fractures and Correlation with Results after Rigid Internal Fixation. *Clin Orthop* **178:7 (1983)**.

Kempf, I., Lootvoet, L., Grosse, A., et al.: Les fractures comminutives de jambe, proposition de classification et étude thérapeutique. *Rev Chir orthop* **58:123 (1972)**. *Rev Chir orthop* **59:43 (1973)**.

Postel, M., Mazas, F., de la Caffinière, J.Y.: Fracture-séparation postérieure des plateaux tibiaux. *Rev Chir orthop, Suppl. 11, 60:317 (1974)*.

Zahlaoui, J., Witvoet, J.: Fractures de jambe. *Encycl Médico-Chirurgicale (Paris)* **14086 A**[10].

43- Heim, U.: Le traitement chirurgical des fractures du pilon tibial. *J Chir (Paris)* **104:307 (1972)**.

44- Florent, J.: Fractures du cou-de-pied. *Encyl Médico-Chirurgicale (Paris)* **14061 C**[10].

Heim, U.: Indications et techniques des sutures ligamentaires dans les fractures malléolaires. *Communication SO.F.C.O.T. XLVIIe Réunion annuelle.*

Lecestre, P., Ramadier, J.O.: Les fractures bimalléolaires et leurs équivalents. *Rev Chir orthop* **62:71 (1976)**.

Weber, B.G.: Die Verletzungen des oberen Sprunggelenks. 2. Auflage. Bern-Stuttgart-Wien: Hans Huber-Verlag 1972.

Glossary = Dictionary

Severity and Complexity

These two terms must be defined at the very beginning as they are frequently used in ortho-paedics interchangeably to denote very different states and conditions.

Severity: The severity of a fracture is used in this book in a specific meaning. For us, the term "severity" implies anticipated difficulties of treatment, the likely complications of treatment, and finally the prognosis.

Complexity: This term is frequently used by traumatologists to describe a combination of a fracture with another lesions, as for instance an open fracture. In this text the term "complex" has a precise meaning. It means a fracture with one or more intermediate fragments in which after reduction there is no contact between the main proximal and distal fragments.

The Classification

The specific terms used in this text provide, when used in the proper sequence, the exact description of the fracture. It is not possible to catalogue by illustration every fracture pattern. It is in the text therefore and not in the illustrations that we find the exact description and definition of a fracture.

location (act of finding the location = localization)
Bone and bone groups are designated by one number: 1 Humerus, 2 Radius/Ulna, 3 Femur, 4 Tibia/Fibula, 5 Spine, 6 Pelvis, 7 Hand, 8 Foot, 9 other bones.
Segments are designated by one number (long bones), two numbers (patella, clavicle, scapula), or three numbers (spine). The three segments for the long bones are: 1 = proximal, 2 = diaphyseal , 3 = distal. For the tibia/fibula, a fourth segment is added, 4 = malleolar.
For the pelvis, the two segments are: 1 = extra-articular, 2 = acetabulum.
For the spine we have three segments: 1 = cervical, 2 = thoracic, 3 = lumbar, which are subdivided into 7, 12 and 5 subsegments.
In segment 9 (other bones), two numbers are designated for the Patella = 1.1, the Clavicle = 1.2, the Scapula = 1.3.

fracture type: In each bony segment, the fractures are divided into three fracture types coded by the letters: A, B, and C.

group: Each fracture type is further subdivided into three groups coded by the numbers: 1, 2, and 3. A group is identified by the combination of the letter representing the fracture type with the corresponding number for the group. Thus there are 9 possible groups for each bone segment. If a fracture does not fit one of these groups, it is classified into a special group denoted by the letter D, e.g. D1.

subgroup: Each group is subdivided into three subgroups coded: .1, .2, and .3. If a fracture does not fit into existing subgroups it is coded as .4.

qualification: Greater precision is added to the classification by adding one of the qualifications. Each qualification adds a further level of precision to the description of the fracture. The qualifications are identified by a code number from 1 to 9 which is placed in parentheses after the number denoting the subgroup. If a qualification applies equally to all the fractures of a group, it appears in the alpha-numerical code immediately after the code for the group (see p. 26 and 184, A2).

Characteristics of Fractures

General Terms:

simple: A term used to characterize a single circumferential disruption of a diaphysis or metaphysis or a single disruption of an articular surface. Simple fractures of the diaphysis or metaphysis are spiral, oblique or transverse.

multifragmentary: A term used to characterize any fracture with one or more completely separated intermediate fragment(s). In the diaphysis and metaphysis it includes the wedge and the complex fractures.

The terms *wedge* and *complex* are used only for diaphyseal or metaphyseal fractures.

wedge: A fracture with one or more intermediate fragment(s) in which after reduction there is some contact between the main fragments. The spiral or bending wedges may be intact or fragmented.

complex: A fracture with one or more intermediate fragment(s) in which after reduction there is no contact between the main proximal and distal fragments. The complex fractures are spiral, segmented or irregular.

comminuted: The term comminuted is imprecise and should not be used.

impacted: A stable and usually simple fracture of the metaphysis or epiphysis in which the fragments are driven one into the other.

center of a fracture: Its determination is pivotal to the assignment of a fracture to a particular bony segment.

simple fracture: the center of the fracture is obvious

198

wedge fracture: the center is at the level of the broadest part of the wedge

complex fracture: the center can only be determined after reduction

severity: A term used to denote the morphologic complexity, the difficulties of treatment and the prognosis of a fracture.

Specific Terms for the Diaphysis:

A – simple: A single circumferential disruption of the diaphysis. Small cortical fragments which represent less than 10% of the circumference are ignored in the classification since they are of no significance for the treatment or prognosis.

Simple fractures of the diaphysis are spiral, oblique or transverse.

A1: *simple spiral*

A2: *simple oblique.* The angle between the fracture plane and a perpendicular to the long axis of the bone is greater than 30 degrees.

A3: *simple transverse.* The angle between the fracture plane and a perpendicular to the long axis of the bone is less than 30 degrees (p. 16).

B – wedge: A fracture of the diaphysis with one or more intermediate fragment(s) in which after reduction there is some contact between the main proximal and distal fragments. Wedge fragments of the diaphysis are:

B1: *spiral wedge*, the so-called butterfly fragment, the result of torsion.

B2: *bending wedge*, a triangular extrusion wedge, the result of bending.

B3: *fragmented wedge*, a wedge fragment which is further fragmented.

C – complex: A fracture with one or more intermediate fragment(s) in which after reduction there is no contact between the main fragments.

Complex fractures of the diaphysis are:

C1: *complex spiral*, a diaphyseal fracture with multiple spiral wedge fragments.

C2: *complex segmental*, a diaphyseal fracture at two levels (bifocal). After reduction the intermediate fragment makes contact with more than 50% of the circumference of each of the main fragments. The intermediate fragment itself can be associated with one or two further wedge fragments. If the intermediate fragment is fragmented, the fracture is classified under C3.

C3: *complex irregular*, a diaphyseal fracture with a number of irregular intermediate fragments.

Specific Terms for the Proximal and Distal Segments:

*Fractures of the proximal and distal segments are either **extra-articular** or **articular**.*

extra-articular: These do not involve the articular surface although they may be intracapsular. They include apophyseal and metaphyseal fractures.

articular: Articular fractures involve the articular surface. They are subdivided into **partial** or **complete.**

partial articular fractures: The fracture involves only part of the articular surface, while the rest of the surface remains attached to the diaphysis.

Types of partial articular fractures:

– **pure split:** A fracture resulting from a shearing force in which the direction of the split is usually longitudinal

– **pure depression:** An articular fracture in which there is pure depression of the articular surface without a split and without separation. The depression may be central or peripheral.

– **split-depression:** A combination of a major split and a depression in which the joint fragments are usually separated.

– **multifragmentary depression:** A fracture in which part of the joint is depressed and the fragments are completely separated

complete articular fractures: The articular surface is disrupted and completely separated from the diaphysis. The severity of these fractures depends on whether its articular or metaphyseal components are simple or multifragmentary.

Anatomy

Humerus:

Condyle of the humerus = the whole distal articular surface of the humerus including the capitellum and the trochlea.

Radius/Ulna:

dorsal = posterior,

volar = anterior,

dorsal rim = description of a partial articular fracture of the distal radius in the frontal plane in which the detached fragment consists of the distal dorsal rim together with a portion of the articular surface (see 23-B2);

volar rim = description of a partial articular fracture of the distal radius in the frontal plane in which the detached fragment consists of the distal volar rim together with a portion of the articular surface (see 23-B3).

Femur:

trochanteric area = part of the proximal segment delineated proximally by the intertrochanteric ridge and distally by a transverse line passing through the inferior edge of the lesser trochanter (see pp. 10 and 56);

subtrochanteric area = part of the diaphysis delineated superiorly by a transverse line passing through the inferior edge of the lesser trochanter medially and distally by a transverse line 3 cm distal to the lesser trochanter.

distal zone of the femoral diaphysis = begins with the flare of the distal femoral diaphysis (see p. 22).

Tibia/Fibula:

intercondylar eminence = tibial spines;

condyles = medial and lateral portions of the proximal segment, each of which supports an articular surface;

anterior tubercle = antero-lateral portion of the distal tibial epiphysis which serves as the area of insertion of the anterior inferior tibio-fibular ligament (tubercle of Chaput);

posterior tubercle = postero-lateral portion of the distal tibial epiphysis which serves as an area of insertion for the posterior inferior tibio-fibular ligament;

syndesmosis = distal tibio-fibular articulation which is maintained by an anterior and a posterior ligament and the interosseous membrane.

Preferred Terms:

dorsal, instead of posterior;

volar, instead of anterior;

supra, instead of above;

infra, instead of below;

comminution / fragmentation = these terms are rarely used in the text as they both convey action and are therefore inappropriate for the description of a static state (e.g. fracture pattern post-injury). Instead fractures are described in specific terms such as "complex, spiral, or fragmented wedge, or complete articular multifragmentary fracture.

U. Heim, Gümligen-Bern; **K. M. Pfeiffer,** Basle

Internal Fixation of Small Fractures

Technique recommended by the AO-Asif Group
Third edition of small fragment set manual

In collaboration with J. Brennwald, C. Geel, R. P. Jakob, T. Rüedi, B. Simmen, H. U. Stäubli

Translated by T. C. Telger

Drawings by K. Oberli

3rd ed. 1988. XI, 393 pp. 258 figs. in more than 700 sep. illus.
Hardcover DM 298,– ISBN 3-540-17728-0

The subject of this book is the operative treatment of small-bone fractures which demand a specially refined instrumentarium and small implants. The emphasis is on articular fractures, particularly in the shoulder girdle, elbow, wrist, hand, talocalcaneal joint and foot, and minor fractures in the area of the knee. The book is intended as a companion volume to the **Manual of Internal Fixation.**

The bulk of the text is concerned with indications and step-by-step technique illustrated in semidiagrammatic figures. Each chapter contains examples of typical clinical radiographs, accompanied in some cases by details of long-term results.

Distribution rights for Japan: Igaku Shoin Ltd., Tokyo

The third edition is scheduled for publication in December 1990:

M. E. Müller, M. Allgöwer, R. Schneider, H. Willenegger

Manual of Internal Fixation

3rd. ed. 1990. Hardcover. ISBN 3-540-52523-8

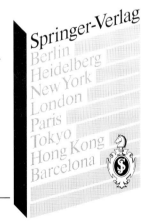

Springer-Verlag
Berlin
Heidelberg
New York
London
Paris
Tokyo
Hong Kong
Barcelona

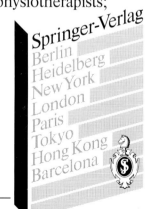